Fraud and Misconduct in Biomedical Research

Fraud and Misconduct in Biomedical Research

Third edition

Edited by

Stephen Lock

Research Associate, Section of the History of Twentieth Century Clinical Science, Wellcome Institute and Editor, British Medical Journal, 1975–91

Frank Wells

Director and Consultant Medical Adviser MedicoLegal Investigations Ltd and Chairman, Ethical Issues Committee, Faculty of Pharmaceutical Medicine

Michael Farthing

Professor of Medicine and Executive Dean, Faculty of Medicine, University of Glasgow, UK

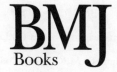

Erratum

Page ix: for Robert Slutsky read William T Summerlin

Chapter 1: superscript reference numbers have been included mistakenly; there are no references for this chapter.

© BMJ Books 2001

First published in 1993
by the BMJ Publishing Group, BMA House,
Tavistock Square, London WC1H 9JR

www.bmjbooks.com

First edition 1993
Second edition 1996
Third edition 2001

British Library Cataloguing in Publication Data
A catalogue record for this book is available from the British Library

ISBN 0-7279-1508-8

Typeset by Newgen Imaging Systems (P) Ltd, Chennai, India

Printed and bound by MPG Books, Bodmin, Cornwall

Contents

Contributors

Jennifer Blunt, Chairman of the North Western Multi-centre Research Ethics Committee, Manchester, UK

Hans Henrik Brydensholt, High Court Judge, Chairman of the Danish Committees on Dishonesty, Denmark

Peter Brock, Vice President, Global Medical Affairs, European Medical Director, Wyeth, Europa, Maidenhead, UK

Jean-Paul Demarez, Cabinet Hardard, Paris

David Edwards, General Practitioner, Lancaster House Medical Centre, London, UK

Stephen Evans, Visiting Professor, Medical Statistics, The London School of Hygiene and Tropical Medicine, UK

Michael Farthing, Professor of Medicine and Executive Dean, Faculty of Medicine, University of Glasgow, UK

C Kristina Gunsalus, Associate Provost, University of Illinois, Illinois, USA

Peter Jay, Chief Executive, MedicoLegal Investigations Ltd, Knebworth, Stevenage, UK

Arthur Horowitz, Principal, Arthur M Horowitz and Associates, Rockeville, Maryland, USA

Jean-Marc Husson, Fondation-Hôpital Saint Joseph, Paris and European Diploma in Pharmaceutical Medicine (Eudipharm), Lyon, France

Marcel C La Follette, Independent Scholar, Washington DC, USA

Veikko Launis, Lecturer in Philosophy, University of Turkey, Department of Philosophy, Finland and Member of the National Research Ethics Council, Finland

Stephen Lock, Editor in Chief, British Medical Journal, 1975–91

Magne Nylenna, Editor in Chief, The Journal of the Norwegian Medical Association, Oslo, Norway

Lesley H Rees, Professor of Chemical Endocrinology and Honorary Consultant Physician, St Bartholomew's and The Royal London School of Medicine and Dentistry, and Director of Education, Royal College of Physicians, London, UK

Drummond Rennie, Institute for Health Policy Studies, University of California San Francisco, USA

Povl Riis, Professor of Medicine, University of Copenhagen, Denmark

Stefanie Stegemann-Boehl, Assistant Head of Division, Federal Ministry for Education, Science, Research and Technology, Berlin, Germany

Frank Wells, Director and Consultant Medical Adviser, MedicoLegal Investigations Ltd, and Chairman, Ethical Issues Committee, Faculty of Pharmaceutical Medicine

Preface to the third edition

By the time this third edition is published, almost thirty years will have elapsed since Robert Slutsky's painted mice inaugurated the paradigm shift into the unthinkable: that misconduct might occur in scientific research. Most authorities now agree that the problem is small but important, yet different countries have reacted in remarkably different ways. Some (the USA and the Nordic countries, in particular) have devised robust and fair systems, honing the details with experience. Others (especially the ancient regimes, such as Britain, France, and Germany) have been less resolute, and hence sometimes individual initiatives have arisen to fill the gap. Two of the latter – a private investigatory agency and a journal editors' organisation – are described here, while other new articles deal with the role of research ethics committees, the experience of a whistleblower, and how to prevent misconduct. The remaining articles, including those detailing the experience of individual countries, have all been updated from previous editions. We are also grateful to Professor Povl Riis for his article putting the entire subject into the wider perspective of scientific research and its relation to society. Two of us (Stephen Lock and Frank Wells) welcome Michael Farthing to the editorial team. His will be the responsibility for taking this book forward into the future.

As before, we have not imposed a straitjacket of terminology on our contributors: fraud, misconduct, dishonesty may all mean the same thing – whatever, Humpty-Dumpty-like, the authors intend. We also have to confess to editorial bias in our approach. Self-evidently, the editors come from a country whose medical Establishment has singularly failed to devise a formal system of prevention and management of a suspected case, despite the continuing evidence that the problem is no different from that in other countries that have taken it seriously. Would that a fourth edition will not need to include again a plea for creating a system in the UK and a few other countries, but can instead be devoted to sharing worldwide experiences of success. However, we remain sceptical.

STEPHEN LOCK
FRANK WELLS
MICHAEL FARTHING
June 2001

Finally it is a pleasure to thank BMJ Books for their continuing help, especially Mary Banks, our indefatigable editor, and Michèle Clarke, the copy-editor.

Preface to the second edition

Events have moved fast since the first edition of this book. In the United States the Office of Scientific Integrity has been replaced by the Office of Research Integrity (ORI), whose newsletters and annual reports show that the system is now dealing with many cases expeditiously and with due process – while seminars and conferences on the topic have been described as a growth industry. In particular, one fear that the courts may assume a more important role has been realised by a successful qui tam suit in May 1995 (though the decision is now under appeal). Feeling that she would get nowhere through the official channels, Pamela Berge, a former Cornell epidemiologist, filed a suit under the False Claims Act alleging that the University of Alabama, Birmingham, had made false claims in its NIH grant application and had used her work on cytomegalovirus. The jury in the Federal District Court found for Berge, stating that the false claims amounted to $550 000; by statute (the article in *Science* – 26 May 1995, p 1125 – states) the UAB is required to pay the government triple that amount, and Berge is entitled to 30% of what the government recovers, as well as $265 000 from the four researchers in compensatory and punitive damages. Elsewhere, several more countries have set up mechanisms to address the issues: Austria and the other Nordic countries now have central committees similar to the Danish one; France is galvanising its drug inspectorate, and Canada is requiring its universities to develop guidelines for handling allegations; and the United Kingdom, criticised in a hardhitting television programme for its inaction – and spurred on by the Pearce case (pages 19 and 252 in the second edition) – is to debate setting up a central committee. There has also been extended interest in the subject even in areas where something was already being done. In the pharmaceutical industry, for example, there has been a flurry of seminars and conferences on the handling of suspected data and there is now a collective agreement by the European industry and the profession to take action against any doctor generating fraudulent data in clinical research. There has also been a concern to extend the scope of the discussion to new topics – in particular, the argument by Iain Chalmers and his colleagues in the Cochrane collaboration that under-reporting of research is another form of misconduct, given that this can lead to seriously misleading recommendations for clinical practice and for new research. Above all, the scientific community is now doing something about the pressing issues of prevention, as shown by *Science's* special feature on everyday dilemmas in research (23 June 1995), the same journal's electronic discussion facility "Science Conduct On-Line", and Chalmers's further proposal that prospective registration of research projects in central registers, possibly founded on research ethics commit-tees, would prevent a lot of non-existent trials from getting published.

To discuss such changes, we asked our contributors to update their chapters when necessary and commissioned some new ones. VandenBurg, Evans, Brock, Hodges, and Gillespie have left their chapters unaltered – whereas Howie, Hosie, Lock, Wells, Riis, Swan, Shapiro, and Maisonneuve have all altered theirs. Among the new contributions La Follette provides the much needed philosophical framework that we had hoped to include in the first edition. Horowitz reviews many of the details of the United States policies and procedures, while Stegemann-Boehl shows how some mechanism might be established in Germany, a country where commentators have claimed that this would be impossible. Finally, Husson and his colleagues extend our knowledge of the European scene, while Altounyan gives an outsider's view based on her extensive research for the BBC "Horizon" programme in March 1995.

"The next book will probably present a structured and systematic description of the disease, its detection, and its management." Would, alas, that this were possible! To be sure, we were encouraged by the largely favourable reviews of our first edition, and have now tried to address some of the constructive points raised by the other reviews, such as the one above. Several critics suggested that the chapters could be ordered more logically, and, though taken together all of the proposed changes would have cancelled one another out, we have now loosely grouped the accounts into history, prevention and management, other aspects, and experience in individual countries.

The most cogent, and consistent, criticism, however, was our failure to define our terms. This problem, however, has perplexed better minds than ours, and significantly it is high on the agenda of the new commission set up by the ORI. The dilemma hinges on a particular difficulty: is fraud solely falsification, fabrication, and plagiarism, or does it extend to "other practices that seriously deviate from those that are commonly accepted within the scientific community" – and even then would it go as far as disciplinary offences, such as sexual harassment? Perhaps what we need are terms to cover different aspects; fraud could then, say, be applied to the most egregious offences, and scientific misconduct or dishonesty (the term used in Denmark) to the entire range, details of which are best specified. For the moment, however, we have stuck to our original title, allowing authors their own choice of words, having ensured that they define these in the first place. Our critics are, of course, entitled to their views, but they should say what words they would prefer, and why.

STEPHEN LOCK
FRANK WELLS
January 1996

PART I
SETTING THE SCENE

1: The concept of scientific dishonesty: ethics, value systems, and research

POVL RIIS

I have been interested in the problem of scientific dishonesty ever since the classic cases occurred in the USA and elsewhere from the mid-1980s onwards, and later with my involvement in the formation of the Danish central committee (undertaken before we had ever had a recent major case in the country). Here, however, I want to take a much broader look at the whole question, in particular trying to put it into the broader context of biomedical ethics.

The three concepts in my subtitle appear all the time in today's publications. Research is, of course, a well-known term; ethics have acquired linguistic citizenship in medicine in the last 30–50 years; but value systems are a "johnny-come-lately" in our vocabulary. Nevertheless, the meaning of each term is often considered self-evident, and all of them are often used with a variety of different connotations. Any discussion of these key concepts in the context of scientific dishonesty needs, then, to start with definitions.

Definitions

Research

Research is defined here[1] as an original endeavour comprising:

- An idea leading to the first ("original") attempt to link two masses of knowledge (already existing or arising out of previous research) with the aim of detecting causal relationships and not merely coincidences.
- The transfer of the idea to one or more precise questions, characterised by the existence of potential answers.
- A bias-controlling methodology intending to link the question(s) to potential answers. (*Methodology* is defined as the art of planning, technically carrying through, interpreting, and publishing scientific research.) Good scientific methodology not only reduces the number of

3

"honest mistakes" within a project, but also makes the research more transparent. Hence it has a preventive effect on the prevalence of scientific dishonesty.

Value systems

Value systems cover all the measures of the non-material qualities of human life. Examples with a special relevance for scientific dishonesty are truth, reliability, responsibility, justice, and freedom. Values may be sub-grouped into *common values* in a society (including those forming the basis of laws) and *individual values*, reflecting value diversity. The latter term is synonymous with *value pluralism* – on the one hand, a welcome part of citizens' freedom; on the other, a potential cause of difficulty (for example, for committees monitoring research ethics or scientific honesty and being faced with value judgments intending to reflect a "social consensus".

If, for instance, a scientific project aiming at evaluating the reliability and risks of preimplantation diagnostic procedures in fertilised human eggs is sent to a research ethics committee, both lay and scientific members might reflect social diversity and not social consensus. Some members might find the method promising, compared with villus biopsy or amniocentesis, because infertile couples could be helped more effectively. Others might find the perspectives frightening because these represent a discrimination against people with malformations or other congenital handicaps.

When values themselves comprise spectra – as, for instance, freedom, justice, and truth – the value universe becomes even wider, and so cut-off points have to be introduced on the value scales. Such cut-off points are called *norms*, a typical example being the term "freedom", defined as the sum of the individual citizen's personal options. In a democratic society, another fundamental value, "justice", needs the application of a norm on the freedom scale: personal freedom has to be limited at a point where any extension would reduce the freedom of other citizens. (In other words, this is a normative cut-off point.)

Ethics

As a term loaded with awe, ethics is often not defined at all, or merely etymologically from its Greek derivation, *ethos*, meaning habits, but, again, to use the term in a serious context, we have to provide a contemporary definition. Here, ethics is defined as:

- The collection of fundamental values, attitudes, and norms considered by most of the population as essential for personal life, life with one another, and life in relation to a society's institutions. Some of these values vis-à-vis biomedical research and national health services are: equality, the Samaritan duty, justice, truth, responsibility, professional competence, and freedom.

- The relation between ethics and the law is bimodal. Ethics, with its fundamental values, forms the basis of legislation. Nevertheless, it also comprises values that are not controlled by the law, but are still decisive elements in societal and personal life.

Value universes of biomedical research

Until recently science had an elite status. Scientists were considered more honest than ordinary citizens, and hence an idea was current that research dishonesty did not occur outside fiction (as in "Dr Jekyll and Mr Hyde"). Today, however, we know better, and so can deal with this aspect in theoretical terms. The value universes of biomedical research concern two main subgroups:

- those related to society in general – the *external universe*;
- those related to the research community itself – the *internal universe*.

The former is concerned with the safety and trust of patients (not only patients in general but also trial patients in particular as well as healthy volunteers).

Thus the first aspect is the ethics of the research so far as the safety of and respect for the citizens acting as subjects are concerned. The evaluation rests primarily with research ethics committees, but the necessary premises also depend on the honesty of the researchers – and hence on knowing the risks to the participants, the potential benefits of the expected results, and an up-to-date survey of the literature.

The second aspect of the honesty/dishonesty concept is how the scientists recruit the trial subjects: do they fairly present all the undisputed facts to potential participants? Thirdly, are the results interpreted totally independently of any sponsors of the research? If the results are untrue for any reason clinicians may be misled in their treatment, even to the extent that the criminal law becomes involved should patients' health or even lives have been endangered. In this way, the societal value universe comes into close and serious contact with research activities.

Within the internal universe, scientists' *curricula vitae* are the most important premise for decisions on grants, academic appointments or promotions, travel to conferences, etc. Here, with the volume of scientific publications as the currency of the research market, any counterfeiting will have the same negative effects as in the monetary sphere. Values such as truth, justice, and responsibility are all at stake. The result may be that honest investigators sometimes lose out, because they have to spend much time on the project. Conversely, the fraudster can recruit patients faster; can work sloppily in the laboratory; or, most seriously, can fabricate the results or be a sleeping partner in several projects, but still an author in all the publications, thereby collecting much of the currency (here represented by authorship and co-authorship).

5

To sum up, the value spectrum of research has an external part orientated towards society, and an internal part orientated towards the research community itself. Courts and laws control the former (with problems owing to the research community's lack of transparency). Independent bodies with experience in research must control the latter, but at the same time must work as society's open eye. In addition, these bodies must extend their interests into the grey zone, between dishonesty and good scientific practice.

Why do scientists transgress?

The motives behind scientists' transgressions of the prevalent norms for our value universes are partly *universal* – in other words, similar to those behind legal and non-scientific moral transgressions – and partly *special* to the competitive research community. The latter aim at changing the ratio between original ideas and the necessary time and effort spent on methodology to obtain more publications for the *curriculum vitae* without any effort or insecurity. In a neighbouring area there is neither frank dishonesty nor good scientific practice. Instead, there are numerous "me too" projects, lacking any originality, good methodological planning, or the risk that the research will be fruitless (because the project ends not with an answer "yes" or "no", but with a "sorry, no answer").

All this is also true for non-legitimate authorship – for instance, the practice (often considered as a right by heads of departments) of adding names to a paper. Again, such behaviour is only partly dishonest, although it is not in accordance with good scientific practice. Nevertheless, both "me too" projects and gift authorship contribute to the still prevalent attitude in too many research units that, "We know best about the good traditions in science, and no outsiders should try to teach us anything new or different." In other words, both these phenomena in the grey zone are moral pollutants at a time when honest scientists and editors are trying to clean up the temple of science.

The other motive encountered in scientific dishonesty is the attempt to reduce the standing of competitors by accusing them of irregularities in their research (a euphemism for dishonesty). This is done either by a direct accusation to a national committee, or, more often, by a campaign of rumour-mongering. The motive is often masked as a profound interest in the purity of science, and, even when the accused has been cleared after a thorough investigation, it often achieves its purpose through the psychological burden placed on the accused, the loss of productive time, and the lingering doubts (reflecting the old saying, "There's no smoke without fire"). This kind of whistleblowing has a different motive from that of the "ideal whistleblower", who is usually a junior hands-on member of the same department of the accused and concerned about apparent irregularities. Competitive, false whistleblowing, conversely, takes place between research scientists equally highly placed in the research hierarchy.

What is the driving force to fraud?

The driving force that unites the motives into active dishonesty varies from a criminal element to more cautious attempts to buy valid currency on the black market (more publications on the CV). For obvious reasons we know very little about these intentions, because sanctions are often taken in proved cases without scientists disclosing their motives. Such a policy of "admit as little as possible" is well known from our ordinary courts of law, but it is a source of wonder how often intelligent people can embark on dishonest research, given that they ought to "know better". My qualified bet is that they know very well about the consequences of such behaviour but think that they are too smart to get detected.[1]

Scientific dishonesty in relation to its nature, prevalence, and consequences

The four classic examples of fraudulent behaviour are fabrication, falsification, plagiarism, and theft. All represent transgression of laws and fundamental values known to the transgressor, and so are closely related to the crimes found in a country's penal code. Hence it is justifiable to speak of a general intention to deceive, whether the transgression is admitted or not when the facts come to light. The consequences of such serious scientific dishonesty are most serious in clinical research dealing with life-threatening diseases, as, for instance, in a recent example of treating disseminated breast cancer with bone-marrow transplantation. An obvious parallel is set by the so-called alternative treatments marketed for serious disease without scientific evidence and directly addressing lay people. Here, however, there has been no professional authorisation of the alternative methods, and hence a mixture of individual conceit and protective group insufficiency leads to a general blamelessness.

The next example of dishonest behaviour among scientists deals primarily with the way research results are evaluated and interpreted, and falls into the subgroup of biomedical ethics labelled "publication ethics". Data archaeology and "cleaning" of results for outliers – in other words, results that, if included, would seriously lower r values and increase P values – occur when scientists work with their raw data. Data massage, or archaeology, mean that scientists apply enough statistical tests until one of them produces a sufficiently low P value, without mentioning this multiple hypothesis testing in the subsequent publication. Such dishonest use of statistics is cognate with the exploitation of mass significance – for example, using a 0.05 level of significance and applying 20 significance tests on related data from the same group of subjects, not realising or forgetting that, by chance, at least one of them will show a P value of < 0.05. If done by an experienced scientist, such a practice will be fraudulent; if done by a tyro, then it can be an honest mistake, caused by a lack of methodological insight.

Another dishonest practice occurs in preparing the manuscript. The authors leave out references that point to previous original research, thereby indicating a spurious personal priority, even if this is not overtly claimed.

These types of scientific dishonesty are probably common but often undisclosed. They can distort results important for patients, and thereby have a societal perspective, but most cases are relevant only for the internal universe – that is, they affect competition between scientists.

Gross slovenliness may affect both the active data collection and the publication process. Examples include not searching the global literature, not testing batches of reagents, not ensuring accuracy of the numerical analyses, or not reading proofs properly and so on. Again, with a young inexperienced scientist such slovenliness might be accepted as venial; honest, but immature and non-professional (though this would not apply to any adviser). For an experienced scientist, however, such behaviour must be characterised as dishonest. It is often related to non-legitimate authorship, as when a senior scientist, often the boss, is a co-author of a paper reporting work that is then shown to have been fraudulent. Here the boss cannot be excused because of not having participated directly in the dishonesty.

Spurious authorship is the inflationary technique mentioned above. It may occur through a chief's supposed prerogative for co-authorship on all the publications coming from the department, or (at the opposite end of the institutional hierarchy) senior scientists may exclude the name of young, legitimate researchers from the article. Often this occurs after the juniors have left the department, with their seniors thinking of them as mere "water-carriers" despite their important contributions.

The same dishonest attitude is shown by authorships as exchangeable currency – for instance, gift authorship, ghost authorship, or barter authorship. Sometimes these take the form of production collectives ("I will make you a co-author if you do the same for me, given that we are not rivals").

Until formal regulations were introduced[2] duplicate publication was frequent, with the double or even more frequent publication of the same data in two different journals, without any cross-reference to the other and without informing the editors. Other examples of inflating *curricula vitae* are the Salami technique (in which data are cut into thin slices and published separately), or the reverse, the Imalas technique, in which one, two, or more cases are added to an already published series without any statement that most of these have been described elsewhere. (Little is added, save another publication for the CV.)

All these examples of dishonest publication ethics overstep the values truth and justice within the internal universe. Very rarely do they have an additional societal perspective, or come to lower public trust in the scientist. The prevalence of such transgressions is unknown, but one study in a national context showed that it was high.[3] The preventive measures detailed below are probably insufficient to eliminate or even reduce the number of non-legitimate authorships. Instead, several other, and more difficult, measures are being introduced, including a demand that authors specify their contribution in detail, while the ultimate decision on who is an author rests with the editor.[4]

The last subgroup of scientific dishonesty is more a matter of etiquette. An example is when a scientist presents the common work of a group to which he or she is a co-worker in slides and talks, but mentions only his or her own name and none of the co-workers. Clearly such practices are an internal matter for the research group, but they are still important because the resulting personal antagonisms waste much time and other research resources.

Common to almost all the disclosed cases of scientific dishonesty (irrespective of their position on the seriousness scale) are the two excuses also heard in our courtrooms: "I thought that everybody did it," and "I didn't know." Both have to be rejected in coming to a verdict, the first because it presupposes a judicial relativism influenced by the number of transgressions, the second because "ignorance of the law" is no excuse.

Good scientific practice (GSP)

Experience from national control systems has shown how important it is to create a new category between full-blown scientific dishonesty and full respect for all the relevant ethical values, a concept called *good scientific practice* (GSP). In this grey zone are the transgressions that cannot be classified as scientific dishonesty but are not GSP. Hence these are referred to as practices "not in accordance with GSP", where GSP represents the national consensus by scientific societies, research councils, independent scientific editors, and the like.[5] In courses for young scientists, this intermediate category can be used to produce examples close to everyday research work. As a result, examples need not be drawn from the full-blown cases of criminal scientific dishonesty, which readily lose their effect because the common reaction is: "I could never become involved in such a scenario."

The social transfer of values

Values ought to underlie academic education, and not be part of any formal curriculum first met in the classroom. In other words, the values behind GSP have deep roots and can be reinforced during scientific training only by being made visible in everyday life. Hence there are several steps in attaining GSP:

• The first step is the visibility and priority given to fundamental human values (truth, reliability, justice, freedom) in children's upbringing. In other words, honest scientific behaviour is not an ethical subspecialty of a profession, but the projection of general ethical constituents onto a professional universe.

- The second step is the visibility of general values within the research society and an accompanying respect for them during daily activity in research institutes and departments. Probably the strongest influence is personal example, and full correspondence between spoken principles and everyday practice. If the head of the department mouths the right views on authorship, but consistently twists them to expect being a co-author of all its publications, then junior researchers find themselves working with double standards.
- The third step is to set up obligatory courses in GSP for all young scientists and would-be specialists. These will catalyse the development of widespread GSP, including the time-consuming change of the traditions of spurious authorship, so that there is a better correlation between scientific productivity and the number of papers in a CV.
- The fourth step is for the controlling body to publish selected cases from the full spectrum of scientific dishonesty in an annual report. And if any word gets out of a possible case before there has been an adjudication, then openness is the keyword. This should not be in the form of details or premature conclusions, but a confirmation that the case does exist with the promise that direct information will be supplied once it has been concluded.

Value conservation and the control of scientific dishonesty

For countries that have had no formally established bodies responsible for managing scientific dishonesty – and even for countries with unofficial mechanisms for examining allegations – it may be valuable to consider the different models and procedures.

The most common set-up is institutional, usually established unprepared and *ad hoc* if an allegation arises in a university or another scientific institution. The initial way of tackling such problems is often an official denial, or at least deep silence. If the case cannot remain in the dark in the long run, then the institution sometimes reacts fiercely with sanctions to show its high moral standards, despite the earlier downgrading of the case. Moreover, interinstitutional distributions of power between involved scientists and the leadership may represent a strong bias against justice. Historically one may apply Montesquieu's triad, demanding that the three components – the legislature, the judiciary, and the executive – should be kept independent of one another. Here, on the contrary, they are mixed to an unacceptable degree.

The alternative to the institutional set-up is the national, or regional, committee. This may be established in two principal ways – either on a legal basis or created by research councils, academies, and scientific societies in common. Further, its remit may be restricted to biomedical research or be extended to cover all kinds, such as the humanities, social sciences, and technical sciences. If such a body deals only with inquiries and investigations, but not with sanctions (which are left to the institutions), at least part of the triad is split into its individual components. If further definitions of scientific dishonesty (or, more importantly of GSP) are promulgated widely, then another step has been taken to secure both the accused and the whistleblowers a high degree of fairness.

Such a structure may, for instance, have the following action levels when a case is raised:

- Suspicion arises locally via a whistleblower or the independent committee's own channels (e.g. through the media).
- The committee decides whether the case should be considered.
- The involved parties are informed and asked for their comments, in accordance with judicial principles.
- If the committee decides on an investigation, an independent specialist group is formed once both parties have accepted the suggested membership.
- The *ad hoc* investigative group's report is open for comment from all the parties, and thereafter is evaluated by the committee. Does the case point to scientific dishonesty, non-accordance with GSP, or to an empty suspicion?
- The conclusion is forwarded to the parties and the institution. The latter decides on sanctions if scientific dishonesty has been substantiated, and reports back to the committee so that any disparity between sanctions taken by different institutions can be minimised.[6]

It may seem strange that scientific dishonesty and fraudulent behaviour within biomedicine have attracted so much attention, whereas very little has been written about ethical transgressions in other scientific disciplines – especially in those where the motives for dishonesty (such as strong competition) would make such behaviour just as feasible as in biomedicine. Nevertheless, few countries have extended their national control system to include all scientific sectors.[7] Given the increasing number of transdisciplinary studies involving medicine and, for instance, the humanities, and often qualitative research disciplines, such an extension should be important not only in an overall scientific perspective but for biomedical research as well.

Finally the preventive value of an independent national or regional committee(s) should be emphasised. Publicity about individual cases has a "vaccination effect" on the research community, but this is enhanced if national and international developments are commented on in a national committee's annual report.[8] The didactic use of concrete cases is easier if it is based on experiences of a national overview rather than on sporadic anecdotes through the media. As I have already mentioned, the cases included in courses for young scientists have a much stronger impact when they originate in concrete – even anonymised – cases from a contemporary spectrum, collected out there in real life.

11

Conclusion

The field of scientific dishonesty has developed from casuistic, often serious, cases 30–40 years ago to a stage where the multitude of different transgressions seems to form a basis for a more systematic analysis of motives and methods. The traditional epidemiological figures – true incidences and prevalences – remain unknown, and are probably not even ascertainable. As the criminological literature shows, individual transgressions can be counted only if disclosed, and the same is true for deviant scientists with a relapsing tendency to act dishonestly in science. Nevertheless, data from the national control systems seem to show that serious cases of fraud and its societal effects are relatively rare.[9]

Instead, the spectrum is dominated by cases with internal perspectives for the research society: spurious authorship, lack of planning with well-defined shares for each member of a project group, and cases with both internal and external (that is, societal) perspectives through dishonest methodology, such as data massage, removal of outliers, and the inflation of originality and personal priorities. The number of reported sensational cases reported worldwide managed by institutions or transferred to the law courts has been too few to indicate that these mechanisms should be widely applied. Instead, such cases have indicated the necessity of establishing independent systems – whether national or regional – based on principles long developed and tested in the common judicial systems. The important first step in creating these is to bring editors of national journals and members of research councils, scientific academies, associations, universities, and scientific societies together, to devise a system that will protect both the accused and the whistleblower against unfair procedures. The aim is to make such values the basis for GSP that is both visible and respected.

Here, with such values – far away from applied statistics, techniques of randomisation, and methods for polymerase chain reactions – the important societal perspective of scientific dishonesty is to be found. Immaterial values such as truth, justice, freedom, responsibility, and many others represent the essential grid that makes the greater society and the scientific one cohere – and to form the necessary trust and reliability to enable citizens to work together, or to depend on each other's information and results. In other words, if a society unofficially accepts that speed limits can be ignored, that tax evasion is a kind of Olympic sport, and that fraudulent receipt of social security is venial, then young scientists will meet the demands of GSP less prepared and less able to be influenced. In these circumstances, the only alternative is to thrust an ungrateful task onto an official body such as a National Committee on Scientific Dishonesty.

2: Regulations on scientific misconduct: lessons from the US experience

DRUMMOND RENNIE, C KRISTINA GUNSALUS

In November 2000, a conference was held in Bethesda, MD, to present research into scientific integrity.[1] The research presented was modest, but the importance of this conference was not in the quality of the research. It lay in the fact that the conference was being held at all. In 1988, one of the authors (DR) had proposed, at a meeting of the National Academy of Sciences (NAS) in Washington, DC, some modest experiments to determine the prevalence of major scientific misconduct.[2] The reasoning behind this idea was that any response should be geared to the prevalence of the problem. The plan was to find out by confidential audit of the data behind published papers the prevalence of the grossest forms of fraud.

The suggestion met with a storm of abuse. The presenter was told that the experiment – which would be confidential and the results never presented except in aggregate, so no individual misdeeds would ever be revealed – would tear the very fabric of science and destroy the delicate web of trust that held scientists together. Yet in 1995, the US Government Commission on Research Integrity made the support of such research one of its key recommendations, and only 12 years after the initial suggestion, this conference took place a few miles from the NAS, co-sponsored by the two great governmental supporters of research, the National Institutes of Health (NIH) and the National Science Foundation (NSF), as well as by the prestigious Association of American Medical Colleges and the American Association for the Advancement of Science. Numerous studies were presented.

The conference was not only oversubscribed, but it passed off without incident and has left science, in the US at least, not merely unscathed, but looking good to the public. Its sponsorship and its reception were powerful indications that, with the passage of time, the US scientific establishment has become less defensive in its attitudes. A month later, in December 2000, the US Government issued a set of revised, government-wide policies on research misconduct, policies that apply equally to all research and researchers, from

13

anthropologists to mathematicians to biologists.[3] Unless you were looking very closely, you would not have noticed this event – an indication of how routine the handling of allegations of research misconduct has already become on this side of the Atlantic.

Contrast this picture with what is happening in the UK. There it is clear that everything is almost exactly 15 years behind the US.[4] As case after case of misconduct blows up in the media, institutional officials scurry around trying to reinvent the wheel in coming up with a response to scientific misconduct, or to cover up the problem.

A memorable meeting, held in Edinburgh in November 1999, at the instigation of medical journal editors, and attended by representatives of important professional societies and journal editors, drew up a consensus statement.[5] To some, action seemed imminent. Yet a year later, three of the editors, in an editorial made up in equal parts of anger, despair, and disgust, pointed out that no official action has occurred and the situation has only become worse.[6] Meanwhile, coverage in the media becomes steadily more intense and the public more disillusioned. Our experience in the US tells us that failure to move in a year is to be expected. What concerns us here is failure to move in 20 years at a time when the happenings in the US over the previous 25 years have scarcely been kept secret from the UK.

When the first cases arose in the US, it was often stated in the UK that this must be a peculiarly American disease, a consequence of the competitive nature of science in the US. However, for years it has been clear that this attitude, which never had evidence to support it, was nonsensical and that scientific misconduct knows no national boundaries. The cases occurring in the UK have not been trivial. Despite that, the paths being followed in the two countries seem to be diverging. In the US, relative calm means relative consensus and, most importantly, reflects effective handling of cases, yet the increasing storminess in the UK could, we believe, have been avoided if the UK had been more able or willing to listen to, and learn from, the massive, well-documented experience gained across the Atlantic.

What happened in the US in the intervening years to bring about the current state of affairs where a new definition can be introduced without controversy? What are the new US Governmental Regulations? How good are they? What lessons do they and this story have for the rest of the world, particularly the UK?

The US experience

A rancorous tone

In the US, the tone that characterised the struggle between scientists and the Federal Government on the issue of scientific misconduct was evident from the start. In 1981, during testimony in the first of over a dozen Congressional hearings, the opening witness, the President of the National Academy of Sciences, asserted that problems were rare – the product

14

of "psychopathic behavior" originating in "temporarily deranged" minds – and called for Congress to focus its attention on increasing the funding for science rather than on these aberrant acts.[7] The Chairman, then-Congressman Albert Gore, Jr, thanked him for this "soothing and reassuring testimony". At the conclusion of the hearing, however, Gore could not "avoid the conclusion that one reason for the persistence of this type of problem is the reluctance of people high in the science field to take these matters very seriously."[8]

This edgy tone characterised practically every step of the process until the first Federal Regulations were issued eight years later, in 1989. It is worth noting that though the regulations were federal, in that they applied equally to researchers and their institutions in every state, until the end of 2000, they still applied officially only to research performed under grants from the Public Health Service (which includes the NIH) and the NSF, which funds much biomedical research. This was presumably because the cases of research misconduct that grip the imagination of the media, the public, and their elected representatives were those involving physicians and clinical research. However, as it was hard for research institutions to operate with more than one set of rules governing misconduct, these early, restricted regulations had a widespread effect. Even later, as general consensus as to handling of cases, standards, and a common, government-wide definition (which *de facto* covers all research conducted at US universities and hospitals) emerged, the process was marked by continuing rancour and heated – and often unsupportable – rhetoric. This aspect of the American experience seems worth understanding, as it may well be impeding progress elsewhere.

Most informed observers agree that serious scientific misconduct is probably quite rare in what is a large and successful scientific enterprise. If that is so, why does the debate about the definition and handling of misconduct arouse so much antagonism? Part of the reason is that hardworking and honest scientists resent the disproportionate attention the media give to occasional spectacular cases of malfeasance, but even those who are resigned to the media's emphasis upon flashy bad news at the expense of workaday good news seem to have felt personal jeopardy from the original proposal to implement rules governing misconduct, and then later from any, and every, proposed change to those rules. A common element seemed to be apprehension that rules would be unfairly applied to one's own solid science. Had the scientific community been deeply divided at any point as to definition and response, this visceral fear would be easier to understand. What is so confusing is that the divisions have been only at the margins, and careful examination of the issues shows a consistent, remarkably high level of general and fundamental agreement throughout the implementation process.

History

In early 1993, we gave a brief account of the turbulent history of scientific misconduct in the US.[9] Until 1989, universities and the Federal Government relied upon *ad hoc* efforts to respond to allegations of malfeasance, much as now seems to be the case in the UK. We described the widespread publicity that accompanied numerous cases in the 1980s and the consequent public perception that fraud was rife. We noted the reaction of the US Congress, which asserted that there was a major problem; and that of research institutions and scientists who, without providing evidence, countered that it was uncommon, and should be left to them to handle. Finally, we noted how the massive publicity and the mishandling of aggrieved whistle-blowers caused Congress to conclude that the institutions' track record was too spotty to maintain the public trust. Despite continuing resistance from scientists and their institutions, Congress insisted on some accountability and governmental oversight, predicated on the government's responsibility to oversee the proper use of tax dollars. The result was the requirement that the main federal funding agencies promulgate regulations and establish offices to provide a more systematic and structured response to allegations of malfeasance.

Definition

The definition adopted in 1989, under Congressional pressure, was "Fabrication, falsification, plagiarism or other practices that seriously deviate from those that are commonly accepted within the scientific community for proposing, conducting, or reporting research."[10]

This definition caused problems for many reasons. Everyone agreed that fabrication, falsification, and plagiarism were antithetical to good science. However, the phrase "... other practices that seriously deviate ..." was immediately seized upon by the Federation of American Societies of Biology (FASEB), who argued that this clause could allow penalties to be applied to novel or breakthrough science, and mobilised its members to remove this phrase completely and limit the definition to "FF&P". As we noted,

Underlying the objections to the "other practices that seriously deviate ..." clause is the fear that the vague language will result in application of a vague and misty standard of misconduct that cannot be known in advance. It seems fundamentally unfair to stigmatize someone for behavior they had no way of knowing was wrong. Unhappily, consideration of cases shows that some of the most egregious behaviors, abuse of confidentiality, for example, are not covered by the FF&P label. We cannot have a definition that implies that this sort of behavior is not wrong. Moreover, since we cannot possibly imagine every scenario in advance, the definition must ensure that perpetrators of acts that are deceptive and destructive to science are not exonerated. If they are, the public and our legislators, applying the standards of common sense, will rightly deride the outcome as nonsensical.[9]

Since the Office of Research Integrity (ORI) – the government office charged with oversight of scientific integrity within biomedicine, the research field controlled by the Public Health Service – never invoked the "other practices ... " clause, but the other large scientific grant-awarding government agency, the National Science Foundation (NSF), did, researchers funded by different government agencies effectively came to be covered by different definitions of research misconduct. In addition, ORI, in a move that was purely administrative, and made to reduce the number and complexity of their formidable backlog of cases, announced that it would not take cases of alleged plagiarism if the authors of a work had been co-authors together, not least because such cases proved singularly awkward to sort out. By definition, ORI asserted, all such cases fell into the category of authorship disputes and would not be examined for the elements of plagiarism. NSF never instituted such a policy, and continued to examine cases where students or co-workers alleged that their contributions had been appropriated by another without cause or attribution. A system in which some can have their complaints examined and others cannot, could not succeed for long.

Intent

Science is a risky enterprise, often requiring much trial and error. No one could possibly undertake scientific experiments if error was construed as misconduct. As Mishkin has pointed out, "Misconduct" in legal parlance means a "wilful" transgression of some definite rule. Its synonyms are "misdemeanour, misdeed, misbehaviour, delinquency, impropriety, mis-management, offense, but *not negligence or carelessness*."[11] Distinguishing error from misconduct requires making a judgment about intent. Whilst scientists are often cowed by this necessity, citizens routinely make them in other settings, most notably in our established criminal justice systems.

It is our opinion that this assessment should be made only at the time of adjudication, after the facts of a case of scientific misconduct have been determined, for example, "words were copied" or "no primary data have been produced." This sequential approach has two salutary effects: first, it reduces the potential that the factual determinations will be obscured by other considerations. The danger otherwise is that – as has frequently happened – a panel's sympathy for the accused ("He's too young, too old, meant well", etc.) interferes with a rigorous analysis of events. Second, this approach introduces proportionality into the response: what, if any, consequence should there be, in light of all the relevant circumstances? This factor is important in the final sense of whether the process "worked" or not – both for participants and for observers.

The scientific dialogue model

Originally, the ORI tried to keep misconduct proceedings in the hands of scientists rather than lawyers. The "scientific dialogue model" they advanced soon came under criticism for being unfair and flawed.[9] Changes were made, and the standards for responding to allegations gradually became more structured and legalistic so that results could withstand scrutiny from administrative tribunals. Defendants, faced by the loss of their livelihoods, hired lawyers to insist on their basic right to fundamental fairness and due process. Most fundamental among these rights are the rights to know and to respond to all evidence to be used against an accused. Unfortunately, these rights were all too easy to overlook while collegiality prevailed ("the scientific dialogue"), and where hard issues were not always faced directly or even-handedly.

The early 1990s: the heat increases

Despite these problems, and the heat they engendered, in February 1993, we concluded on a note of cautious optimism:

> ... practically everything to do with scientific misconduct is changing rapidly: the definition, the procedures, the law and our attitudes ... It will take time to accumulate a body of experience (a case law, as it were) and to get it right. The challenge is to seize the opportunity, to capitalize on the wealth of accumulating information, and to focus on the long-term goals of strengthening science and the society that depends on it.[9]

Our optimism was premature. In 1994, despite more than 20 years of widely publicised cases of misconduct, more than a dozen congressional hearings, years of regulations as a result of congressional impatience with science (and layers of modifications to them), and, first, an Office of Scientific Integrity and then of Research Integrity, there remained widespread division and dismay. The definition was still hotly debated, as was the process owed an accused scientist, the extent of federal oversight, how to protect whistleblowers, and how to prevent misconduct. At the same time, in the early 1990s, several high-profile cases were decided against government science agencies and their ways of proceeding.[12]

The Commission on Research Integrity (Ryan Commission) (Figure. 2.1)

In 1993, as part of the Act that continued funding for the National Institutes of Health (NIH), the US Congress mandated the formation of a Commission, charged with considering the whole field, from the definition of misconduct, through the process of handling cases, to whistleblower protection. The Commission, of which the two of us were members, held 15 open meetings in five different cities across the US, and heard hundreds of witnesses "including scientists, whistleblowers, attorneys, institutions, scientific organizations, the press, interested citizens and government officials."[12] The number and severity of the cases presented to the Commission was impressive.

At the end of 1995, asserting that the US Federal Government had an interest in professional misconduct involving the use of federal funds in research and which could affect the public health, the Commission recommended that the definition of research misconduct (Figure 2.1) should be "based on the premise that research misconduct is a serious

1. Commission on Research Integrity's Definition[12]

Research misconduct is significant misbehavior that improperly appropriates the intellectual property or contributions of others, that intentionally impedes the progress of research, or that risks corrupting the scientific record or compromising the integrity of scientific practices. Such behaviors are unethical and unacceptable in proposing, conducting, or reporting research or in reviewing the proposals or research reports of others.

Examples of research misconduct include but are not limited to the following:
Misappropriation: An investigator or reviewer shall not intentionally or recklessly a. plagiarize, which shall be understood to mean the presentation of the documented words or ideas of another as his or her own, without attribution appropriate for the medium of presentation; or b. make use of any information in breach of any duty of confidentiality associated with the review of any manuscript or grant application.

Interference: An investigator or reviewer shall not intentionally and without authorization take or sequester or materially damage any research-related property of another, including without limitation the apparatus, reagents, biological materials, writings, data, hardware, software, or any other substance or device used or produced in the conduct of research.

Misrepresentation: An investigator or reviewer shall not with intent to deceive, or in reckless disregard for the truth, a. state or present a material or significant falsehood; or b. omit a fact so that what is stated or presented as a whole states or presents a material or significant falsehood.

2. Other Forms of Professional Misconduct
a. Obstruction of Investigations of Research Misconduct
The Federal Government has an important interest in protecting the integrity of investigations in reported incidents of research misconduct. Accordingly, obstruction of investigations of research misconduct related to federal funding constitutes a form of professional misconduct in that it undermines the interests of the public, the scientific community, and the Federal Government.

Obstruction of investigations of research misconduct consists of intentionally withholding or destroying evidence in violation of a duty to disclose or preserve; falsifying evidence; encouraging, soliciting or giving false testimony; and attempting to intimidate or retaliate against witnesses, potential witnesses, or potential leads to witnesses or evidence before, during, or after the commencement of any formal or informal proceeding.

b. Noncompliance with Research Regulations
Responsible conduct in research includes compliance with applicable federal research regulations. Such regulations include (but are not limited to) those governing the use of biohazardous materials and human and animal subjects in research.

Serious noncompliance with such regulations after notice of their existence undermines the interests of the public, the scientific community, and the Federal Government, and constitutes another form of professional misconduct.

Figure 2.1   The US Commission on Research Integrity's definition of research misconduct.

violation of the fundamental principle that scientists be truthful and fair in the conduct of research and the dissemination of its results."[12] The Commission, which we will hereafter in this section call "we", strongly recommended the development of a common federal definition of research misconduct and other forms of professional misconduct related to research. With its definitions, we put forward examples within the report (Figure 2.1).

By defining the central terms used in the definition of misconduct, we obviated the problem endemic in institutional proceedings in which every investigative panel secured a dictionary and defined for itself key elements upon which its findings depended. This common and understandable impulse all too frequently compromised the integrity of individual misconduct proceedings, as the resulting *ad hoc* definitions did not pass the "laugh", let alone the "red-face", test. In addition to providing a fuller internal definition of plagiarism, our proposed definition explicitly addressed other issues upon which faculty review panels repeatedly stumbled. For example, we incorporated misconduct in reviewing manuscripts or grant applications into the definition of offenses outside acceptable professional conduct.

We also researched and then recorded the legal reality in the US that the "standard of proof" required in civil proceedings is the "preponderance of the evidence", not the higher standards of "clear and convincing" or "beyond a reasonable doubt". These issues had derailed many an institutional proceeding and prevented them from reaching a finding. Another very important component of the Ryan Commission's work was the declaration that, whilst intent should be a necessary requirement for a finding of fabrication or falsification, a finding of carelessness suffices to support a finding of plagiarism.

We broadened the definition beyond the then-prevailing standard of "fabrication, falsification and plagiarism" to include other forms of unethical behaviour not then governed by any specific regulations (Figure 2.1). Guided by actual cases, we defined research misconduct as:

1 misappropriation (including plagiarism);
2 interference (for example, tampering with someone else's research), and
3 misrepresentation.

In addition, we included categories of lesser misconduct that, whilst not "scientific misconduct", still warranted response. These included:

- obstruction of misconduct investigations;
- retaliation against those participating in investigations, and
- non-compliance with research regulations.

We recognised that, although research institutions might make their own rules, the governmental definition had, after 1989, become *de facto* the one in general use.

In our report, we did not merely list bad acts, but laid out the rights and responsibilities of scientists. We recommended that educational programmes on research integrity should be required in institutions receiving federal money. We wanted:

- to assure that information about good professional conduct be provided as a fundamental element of education;
- to make discussion of these matters more common and less threatening;

- to make it possible for the powerless to ask questions, and
- to make it harder for the clever sociopath to slide by.

We recommended that there be "Funding for scholarship, teaching, and research in science ethics. Such funded research should include an experimental audit of the prevalence of data misrepresentation." We also recommended that "professional societies each adopt a code of ethics in research" and initiate "activities that will further promote the ethical conduct of research and professionalism in science."

Recognising that whistleblowers provide an important quality control mechanism in science, and mindful of the numerous examples of abuse of whistleblowers who had brought forward well-founded allegations, we set forth a detailed appendix to the report *Responsible whistleblowing: a whistleblower's bill of rights* (Figure 2.2). We spelled out the rights and responsibilities of whistleblowers, of the accused and of their institutions. Institutions should deal with "retaliation against whistleblowers as rigorously at the inquiry, investigation, and adjudication stages as they do in cases with research and other professional misconduct"; and that institutions that performed competent investigations should be protected from adverse use of their findings in litigation.[12]

Our Commission made a number of recommendations, based upon our collective experience, the testimony presented at our meetings, our research, and information presented by commissioned papers, about how misconduct proceedings should be conducted. For example, we advised that investigation and subsequent adjudication should always be separated organisationally; that "legal, law-enforcement, and scientist-investigator staff participate in each federally conducted investigation and ensure that scientists participate in hearings and appeal procedures"; that "those conducting investigations have subpoena power over persons and documents"; and that "authorship or collaborative" disputes (those previously dismissed by the Office of Research Integrity, for administrative reasons) should be addressed by institutions and by federal funding agencies.

While our proposals protected institutional decisions from second-guessing, if properly conducted, they recognised the built-in conflicts that institutions can face when investigating their own scientists, some of whom might be influential and bring in large amounts of money. We proposed "widespread, systematic public disclosure of all outcomes of federal research and research-related professional misconduct cases, with detailed, specific statements of their rationale, in view of the strong public interest in the disclosure of information underlying such cases."[12]

We articulated the elements required for fair process, by articulating the various interests at stake in these proceedings – including those of the accused, whistleblowers, witnesses, and funding agencies. We recommended internal checks and balances throughout, even for the federal agencies providing the funding for research. We suggested approaches for streamlining processes, made numerous recommendations to improve the

a. *Communication*: Whistleblowers are free to disclose lawfully whatever information supports a reasonable belief of research misconduct as it is defined by PHS policy. An individual or institution that retaliates against any person making protected disclosures engages in prohibited obstruction of investigations of research misconduct as defined by the Commission on Research Integrity. Whistleblowers must respect the confidentiality of sensitive information and give legitimate institutional structures an opportunity to function. Should a whistleblower elect to make a lawful disclosure that violates institutional rules of confidentiality, the institution may thereafter legitimately limit the whistleblower's access to further information about the case.

b. *Protection from retaliation*: Institutions have a duty not to tolerate or engage in retaliation against good-faith whistleblowers. This duty includes providing appropriate and timely relief to ameliorate the consequences of actual or threatened reprisals, and holding accountable those who retaliate. Whistleblowers and other witnesses to possible research misconduct have a responsibility to raise their concerns honorably and with foundation.

c. *Fair procedures*: Institutions have a duty to provide fair and objective procedures for examining and resolving complaints, disputes, and allegations of research misconduct. In cases of alleged retaliation that are not resolved through institutional intervention, whistleblowers should have an opportunity to defend themselves in a proceeding where they can present witnesses and confront those they charge with retaliation against them, except when they violate rules of confidentiality. Whistleblowers have a responsibility to participate honorably in such procedures by respecting the serious consequences for those they accuse of misconduct, and by using the same standards to correct their own errors that they apply to others.

d. *Procedures free from partiality*: Institutions have a duty to follow procedures that are not tainted by partiality arising from personal or institutional conflict of interest or other sources of bias. Whistleblowers have a responsibility to act within legitimate institutional channels when raising concerns about the integrity of research. They have the right to raise objections concerning the possible partiality of those selected to review their concerns without incurring retaliation.

e. *Information*: Institutions have a duty to elicit and evaluate fully and objectively information about concerns raised by whistleblowers. Whistleblowers may have unique knowledge needed to evaluate thoroughly responses from those whose actions are questioned. Consequently, a competent investigation may involve giving whistleblowers one or more opportunities to comment on the accuracy and completeness of information relevant to their concerns, except when they violate rules of confidentiality.

f. *Timely processes*: Institutions have a duty to handle cases involving alleged research misconduct as expeditiously as is possible without compromising responsible resolutions. When cases drag on for years, the issue becomes the dispute rather than its resolution. Whistleblowers have a responsibility to facilitate expeditious resolution of cases by good faith participation in misconduct procedures.

g. *Vindication*: At the conclusion of proceedings, institutions have a responsibility to credit promptly – in public and/or in private as appropriate – those whose allegations are substantiated.

Every right carries with it a corresponding responsibility. In this context, the Whistleblower Bill of Rights carries the obligation to avoid false statements and unlawful behavior.

Figure 2.2   Responsible whistleblowing: a Whistleblower's Bill of Rights.[12]

effective oversight of institutional performance, and broadened the array of sanctions that could be applied against those found guilty of misconduct, and against institutions failing to carry out investigations properly.

The Reaction

Although the Commission's report was characterised by a disinterested observer, the editor of *The Lancet*, as "a superb piece of analysis",[13] and many academics pronounced themselves content with the commission's definition,[14] it met with widespread condemnation by the scientific establishment. The Commission consisted largely of scientists (as well as ethicists, administrators, and lawyers), but the reaction from the scientific elite in the US was immediate, loud, defensive, dismissive, confused, and self-contradictory. Given that the reaction was in response to a careful report based on the articulated "fundamental principle that scientists should be truthful and fair in the conduct of research and the dissemination of research results," this reaction seemed at times hysterical. The President of the Federation of American Societies for Experimental Biology (FASEB) wrote to the Secretary for Health and Human Services that the "Commission's report is so seriously flawed that it is useless as a basis for policy making and should be disavowed ... We find the definition to be unworkable, and therefore unacceptable."[15] He was quoted in the press as calling the report "an attack on American science".[13] The same letter objected to what was called an expansion of the definition of plagiarism, even though the Commission had been guided in its definition by the Academy's own report, *Responsible science*,[16] a report the latter strongly endorsed.

The NAS leadership also wrote a letter criticising the Commission report. Whilst acknowledging that the Commission "repeatedly states that the primary investigative responsibility rests with the research institutions",[17] it brushed these statements aside in raising the bogeyman of a vast expansion of an intrusive federal bureaucracy, if the Commission's recommendations were to be implemented. The NAS nowhere acknowledged that it was the abject failure of many research institutions to respond appropriately to allegations of misconduct that led to the Commission's original formation by the Congress. The NAS failed to say that the report called only for government agencies to investigate allegations in certain very limited circumstances: in cases involving more than one institution, or where the institution had not conducted a proper investigation.[18] Nor did it note that the government already had such an oversight role, which would, if anything, be diminished if the commission's recommendations were followed.

In hindsight, what was most threatening in the Commission Report was the *Whistleblower's Bill of Rights*.[12] The Commission was accused of failing to "protect adequately the rights of scientists who are accused of misconduct." Yet what moved the Commission was not the rights of scientists who were accused, who already had excellent protections, but the plight of accusers, who blew the whistle in good faith, and who were later proved right, but who suffered considerable harm, often from the guilty and their institution. The Commission had heard testimony from a great many in this position.

Perhaps the most persistent, extraordinary and revealing criticism ·of the report, and, indeed, of any proposed regulation, was the continuing allegation that regulation would impede scientific progress, because truly original science might easily be labelled misconduct. In hundreds, even thousands of cases, this has never happened.

Finally some scientists still claimed that, because science is "self-correcting", no rules were necessary. The corollary of this position is that it doesn't matter if the record is never put right. In the medical field alone, however, the truth is that much science is never replicated, and this assertion says nothing about the costs – institutional and human – imposed by gross fraud, nor the abuse of, and loss of morale among, co-workers, the anger on the part of the public and politicians, and the outrage of the media.

Our report grew out of the failures of the past, including the failure of the 1989 government definition to stand up to legal challenge and to work effectively when applied to real cases. The vehemence of the reaction to the report, which proposed that scientists should be truthful and fair, and which was crafted to make it work in the real world of research and of lawyers, was telling. So was its widespread misrepresentation. Upon reflection, we conclude that this must stem from the fact that few of the scientists who objected had much experience in dealing with allegations of misconduct. Together, they suggest that scientists continue to feel threatened by the spectre that malicious allegations might be brought against them. Above all, objecting scientists failed to grasp the fact that, in this real world, legal challenges dominate the field, and that, in response to these realities, the Ryan Commission introduced precision – which in turn provides protections for those involved in misconduct proceedings, most especially the accused scientist.

We have presented this aspect of the US response in some detail because these sorts of reaction to any regulation may be predicted in the UK, given the striking similarities between the Ryan Commission's "fundamental principle" (above) and the Edinburgh Consensus definition of misconduct as "behaviour that … falls short of good ethical and scientific standards." (see Figure 2.4)[5]

While more than a year has passed since the Edinburgh meeting, it is also worth noting that five years passed from the delivery of the Ryan Commission report until the most recent – and non-controversial – US government regulations.

The US Government-wide Regulations of December 2000 (Figure 2.3)[3]

During the ensuing five years, cases occurred and were reported in the media, and were summarised in regular reports from the ORI and the

Federal Policy on Research Misconduct[a]
I. Research[b] Misconduct Defined
Research misconduct is defined as fabrication, falsification, or plagiarism in proposing, performing, or reviewing research, or in reporting research results.
- Fabrication is making up data or results and recording or reporting them.
- Falsification is manipulating research materials, equipment, or processes, or changing or omitting data or results such that the research is not accurately represented in the research record.[c]
- Plagiarism is the appropriation of another person's ideas, processes, results, or words without giving appropriate credit.
  Research misconduct does not include honest error or differences of opinion.

II. Findings of Research Misconduct
A finding of research misconduct requires that:
- There be a significant departure from accepted practices of the relevant research community; and
- The misconduct be committed intentionally, or knowingly, or recklessly; and
- The allegation be proven by a preponderance of evidence.

---

[a] No rights, privileges, benefits or obligations are created or abridged by issuance of this policy alone. The creation or abridgment of rights, privileges, benefits, or obligations, if any, shall occur only upon implementation of this policy by the Federal agencies.
[b] Research, as used herein, includes all basic, applied, and demonstration research in all fields of science, engineering, and mathematics. This includes, but is not limited to, research in economics, education, linguistics, medicine, psychology, social sciences, statistics, and research involving human subjects or animals.
[c] The research record is the record of data or results that embody the facts resulting from scientific inquiry, and includes, but is not limited to, research proposals, laboratory records, both physical and electronic, progress reports, abstracts, theses, oral presentations, internal reports, and journal articles.

The term "research institutions" is defined to include all organizations using Federal funds for research, including, for example, colleges and universities, intramural Federal research laboratories, Federally funded research and development centers, national user facilities, industrial laboratories, or other research institutes. Independent researchers and small research institutions are covered by this policy.

Figure 2.3   Federal policy on research misconduct.[3]

NSF. Gradually, as the media, the public and the profession realised that the system was working in a routine and reasonably efficient manner, the heat died down, meanwhile, the administration embarked on the lengthy process of making common regulations that would govern all types of research, and not just those in biomedicine.

On 6 December 2000, after a two-month public comment period, the Clinton administration issued the new, government-wide regulations defining research misconduct and laying down the rules for investigation and adjudication of allegations of misconduct concerning research done with US federal funds.[3] Since all important universities and research institutions receive such funds, these regulations will become institutional rules, although institutions are allowed to have their own additional rules if they wish to impose a higher internal standard.

We strongly believe they should, and we say this because the new definition, confining itself to "fabrication, falsification, or plagiarism in proposing, performing, or reviewing research, or in reporting research results," leaves out many actions that we find destructive of good science, and which are not covered by other laws. We were both involved in assessing one case in which a junior investigator had sequestered data and materials from her colleagues – an action that would not be judged to be scientific or research misconduct by the new regulations, though commonsense would tell us that the investigator's conduct in the performance of research was wrong. We are troubled, then, that by making the definition too narrow, other egregious behaviours might seem to be condoned. It would send the worst possible signal if the academic community were to think such behaviour – by default – to be acceptable.

This new definition is again appropriately silent on prolonged non-compliance with other research regulations, such as the unethical treatment of human research subjects or mistreatment of laboratory animals used in research, because there are already regulations governing these problems. Again, the new regulations do not supersede criminal or other civil laws that have nothing to do with the faithful reporting of good science (for example, laws on sexual harassment).

Like the Ryan Commission Report, from which the new rules drew extensively, from the incorporation of interior definitions of critical terms and of states of mind for offences, to articulation of necessary procedural safeguards, the new rules provide the rationale for all the proposals. We strongly recommend that anyone interested in the formulation of adequate institutional responses to allegations of research misconduct, read both the Ryan Commission Report and these new US Government Regulations of December 2000.

Lessons from the US experience

It took 20 years to achieve a set of widely accepted regulations in the US. In the hope that examination and understanding of this experience might prevent a great deal of reinvention of wheels, we will summarise what we believe are the essential elements. First, however, consider the *catalysts*:

- Repeated, dramatic incidents resulting in publicity showing that research institutions operated in ignorance, denial, and cover-up; and there was recurrent shaming of institutions in the media. (This is the present position in the UK.)
- A few powerful politicians, highly sceptical of the establishment's reassurances that all was well, repeatedly exposing the thinness of these reassurances, pushing for regulation, and, finally, exasperated by the "do-nothing" approach of science, forcing regulation to be tied to the continuance of federal research funds. (This is not happening in the UK,

where, in a vacuum, the role has been, to some extent, taken over by a few courageous and outspoken medical editors, starting with Stephen Lock [*BMJ*] and continuing with Richard Smith [*BMJ*], Richard Horton [*Lancet*] and Michael Farthing [*Gut*], with COPE (Committee on Publication Ethics); and by Frank Wells and his notable efforts with the investigation of cases of misconduct in clinical research.)

- Numerous meetings attended by representatives of science, lawyers, administrators, and legislators.
- The establishment of oversight offices predicated on the assumption that research misconduct was basically a clinical research problem. Followed by a gradual realisation that misconduct can occur in every branch of research, from mathematics to the humanities, and that administering its regulations would be much easier if all researchers were governed by the same rules.
- Learning from experiment and hard experience. The "scientific model" did not work when the unfairness and illegality of the process was exposed (usually by lawyers or journalists). Scientists had to learn that processes for appeal were necessary, and that investigation and adjudication should be separated. Gradually a case law built up, and the process was absorbed into those of administrative law.[19-21]
- Greater education all round. Everyone concerned came to realise that it is beneficial to assure that students – no matter who their mentor – receive certain baseline information about good practice, and that, because scientists were mortals, it made sense to have processes in place to deal efficiently and routinely with those who strayed.

Constantly retarding the process of reform are several factors. Many distinguished scientists cannot accept that scientific misconduct can occur until it happens near them and they have to deal with it. More generally, it seems to be a human trait to seek power without accountability, so scientific organisations can be expected to oppose all regulation, including any amendment to even previously-condemned regulations.

Conditions/criteria necessary for any workable system

It must:

- **Be universal.** Across all research disciplines and not confined to clinical research.
- **Be official and published.** The rules must be promulgated by some official and widely accepted body having the legal power to make them stick, and these rules must be published.
- **Have a clear and specific definition.** With internal descriptions of the critical elements.
- **Have a clear and fair process.** Essential elements include:
  - *Notice* to those accused of the charges against them.

27

- *Opportunity to respond to the charges* and to all evidence used to draw conclusions.
- *Opportunity to have an advocate or representative* accompany all those participating in official proceedings (including those accused, those serving as witnesses, and those bringing allegations).
- *Appropriate powers in those charged with performing investigations* to have access to all relevant evidence and witnesses. An investigation cannot stand if those charged with establishing relevant facts do not have full access to all relevant evidence and witnesses. This may require subpoena power.
- *Separation of investigation and adjudication* (that is, those who perform investigations and make findings of fact should be separated from those who judge the totality of the case and impose sanctions).[12,19]
- *Meaningful consequences* for those who violate standards, institutions that countenance misconduct, and for any form of retaliation against those who, in good faith, raise questions about the propriety of scientific conduct.
- *Must allow appeals.* After a proceeding is complete, there must be one opportunity to seek review of the procedures and fundamental fairness employed in reaching the conclusions.

The Joint Consensus Report of 1999 Statement (Figure 2.4)[5]

We have discussed the enormous importance of exact definition, if the process adopted is to be fair and acceptable, since it is obviously unfair for any scientist to be accused of misconduct if there is no clear statement of what constitutes misconduct. Indeed, a basic foundation of the rule of law is that the laws should be specific and published. The Edinburgh Consensus conference was a very important step in beginning to address the problem in the UK, but when we apply our criteria to the definition in the Consensus Statement (Figure 2.4) we find it wanting.

What is good about it?

It recognises that every case of scientific misconduct weakens our trust in science. It also mentions that it goes beyond "FF&P", which we believe to be important, and it recognises that changes may be necessary in the future.

And what is bad?

The Consensus Report is an early stage in an evolutionary process that will probably take years, so it is unfair to criticise it severely, but it is worthwhile to note its deficiencies because they help to tell us what needs to be done.

Was it universal?

The composition of the Consensus meeting, which was largely made up of people interested in clinical research, seemed to suggest a role for the

---

Consensus Statement (Preamble and Definition only)

Patients benefit not only from good quality care but also from good scientific research. We all expect high standards of scientific and medical research practice. The integrity, probity, skill and trustworthiness of scientific and medical researchers are essential if public confidence is to be assured. In the design and execution of biomedical and healthcare research, public participation is essential. The Joint Consensus Conference on Misconduct in Biomedical Research was convened in order to debate, address and offer guidance on key questions because "every single case [of fraud and misconduct] reduces public confidence, abuses the use of public and charitable funds, and causes insult and frustration to the vast majority of careful, honest workers".[1]

The definition of research misconduct

Behaviour by a researcher, intentional or not, that falls short of good ethical and scientific standards

No definition can or should attempt to be exhaustive. It should allow for change. The definition should not be read as being restricted to fabrication, falsification of data and plagiarism. It is intended to cover the whole range of research misconduct.

[1] Rennie D, Evans I, Farthing MJG, Chantler C, Chantler S, Riis P. Dealing with research misconduct in the UK [and other articles]. *BMJ* 1998;**316**:1726–33.

Figure 2.4 Joint Consensus Conference on Misconduct in Biomedical Research 28–29 October 1999.

General Medical Council. However, a proposal that the General Medical Council serve as the fulcrum of a UK system fails the test of universality. As in the US, concern first started when misconduct was found in clinical research, which, of course, seems rather too close to home for most people. But it is a widespread problem. An organisation established to discipline physicians cannot realistically police scientific misconduct when, even in clinical research, most projects involve numerous co-workers with different degrees and expertise, some of them completely outside medicine. Some mechanism must be found to broaden the scope of regulation and enforcement.

Was it official?

The Edinburgh Consensus Report, developed as it was in a closed meeting, even though a good start, and even though it was immediately published, was not issued by any body with the mandate and legal power to make its recommendations happen. Nor was it developed with a broadly-based enough input to build sufficient understanding to produce a result that will be widely accepted.

The *definition* of research misconduct proposed by the 1999 Joint Consensus Conference is neither specific nor does it provide clear guidance on the meaning of its critical terms. Indeed, it is so vague, non-specific, and all-encompassing, that it is unworkable. What are "good ethical standards"? In which field? In what circumstances? By whose judgment? There are whole areas of research – for example, research on stem cells, or on aborted fetuses – where ethical scientists hold strongly divergent opinions about "good" standards. Worst of all, the definition includes unintentional behaviour that falls short of good scientific standards. To give an example, one of us (DR) used to conduct physiologic experiments at high altitude in Nepal. Once a whole batch of specimens was ruined because DR had not known that dry ice would be unavailable during a religious holiday. As a result, the results obtained were incomplete and the differences not statistically significant. I had not met the "good scientific standards" set out clearly in my protocol, devised with my colleagues in the US. If this sort of thing is misconduct, as it clearly would be under this strange definition, how could anyone ever dare to attempt science? In addition, the statement that the definition "is intended to cover the whole range of research misconduct" is circular.

As to "clear and fair process", though the specifics of handling accusations of misconduct are essential ingredients of any successful system, the Consensus Report says little or nothing specific about procedures, so most of the elements necessary for a useful system are undefined or absent. The US experience illustrates that getting the process right matters as much as having the right definition. In fact, one could posit that the low-key acceptance of the new government definition in 2000 is rooted as much in the growing comfort that proceedings – if never pleasant – are not unfair or biased by design. Much can be learned from the American experience with process, both by those with institutional responsibilities, and those who are caught in a specific situation.[19–21]

Conclusion

Some bullfighters in Spain routinely shave the horns of the bulls they face – sometimes by as much as 2.5 cm – to reduce their risk of injury, as it impairs the weapons, vision, and balance of the bull. It is well known this occurs, and it is regarded as wrong, but when the Spanish government proposed a system of examinations to detect irregularities, the bullfighters went on strike, saying that they should be trusted to regulate themselves.[22] We should all like our professions to behave in a way that to most of us would define professionalism, that is, to regulate ourselves effectively, but our experience with scientific misconduct in the US, and the experience with physicians in the UK, shows us that, as with bullfighters in Spain, there must be some higher body to force regulation upon them. We can expect that nothing much will happen in the UK until that fact is absorbed by all concerned, and this will not occur until the pain and shame of bad publicity becomes unbearable.

Meanwhile, no one can expect to draw up regulations in a couple of days, and full of holes as it is, the Edinburgh Statement is a start. Now, using the Ryan Report and the US Federal Regulations, and paying attention to the long and carefully examined experience gathered in the US, as well as to the experience gleaned from other countries (for example, the Scandinavians), we would suggest that the UK begin the hard, contentious but necessary work of framing their own rules. We wish them luck.

References

1 Office of Research Integrity. *A Research Conference on Research Integrity*. 18–20 November 2000, Bethesda, Maryland, USA.
2 Rennie D (ed), Mark, Dupe, Patsy, Accessory, Weasel, Flatfoot. Presentation before the Conference on Ethics and Policy in Scientific Publication. October 1988, National Academy of Sciences, Washington, DC. In: *Ethics and policy in scientific publication*, Washington: CBE, Inc., 1990.
3 Office of Science and Technology Policy, Executive Office of the President. *Federal policy on research misconduct*. Federal Register 6 December 2000, pp. 76260–4. *http://frwebgate.access.gpo.gov/cgi-bin/getdoc.cgi?dbname=2000_register&docid=00-30852-filed* (accessed 10 February 2001).
4 Rennie D. *Why is action needed?* Joint Consensus Conference on Misconduct in Biomedical Research. Royal College of Physicians of Edinburgh, 28 October 1999.
5 Joint Consensus Conference on *Misconduct in Biomedical Research Statement*. 28–29 October 1999. *www.rcpe.ac.uk/esd/consensus/misconduct_00.html*
6 Farthing M, Horton R, Smith R. UK's failure to act on research misconduct. *Lancet* 2000; **356**:2030.
7 Fraud in Biomedical Research. 1 April 1981, Committee on Science and Technology, Subcommittee on Investigation and Oversight. (Statement of Dr Philip Handler, President of the National Academy of Sciences, P10–14.)
8 Fraud in Biomedical Research. 1 April 1981, Committee on Science and Technology, Subcommittee on Investigation and Oversight. P24.
9 Rennie D, Gunsalus CK. Scientific misconduct. New definition, procedures and office – perhaps a new leaf. *JAMA* 1993;**269**:915–17.
10 Public Health Service. Responsibilities of awardee and applicant institutions for dealing with and reporting possible misconduct in science: final rule. *Federal Register* 1989;**54**: 32446–51.
11 Mishkin B. The investigation of scientific misconduct: some observations and suggestions. *New Biologist* 1991;**3**:821–3.
12 *Integrity and misconduct in research. Report of the Commission on Research Integrity** to the Secretary of Health and Human Services, the House Committee on Commerce, and the Senate Committee on Labor and Human Resources. 3 November 1995. *http://gopher.faseb.org/opar/cri.html* (accessed 28 January 2001) (*Ryan Commission).
13 Goodman B. Scientists are split over finding of Research Integrity Commission. *The Scientist* (22 January) 1996:1.
14 Kaiser J. Commission proposes new definition of misconduct. *Science*. 1995;**269**:1811.
15 Ralph A. Bradshaw to Secretary of Health and Human Services Donna Shalala. 4 January 1996: P1.
16 National Academy of Sciences, National Academy of Engineering, and Institute of Medicine. *Responsible science: ensuring the integrity of the research process Vols 1 and 2*. Washington: National Academy Press, 1992.
17 Letter from the National Academy of Sciences Council to William Raub. 15 March 1996.
18 Ryan KJ. Scientific misconduct in perspective: the need to improve accountability. *Chronicle for Higher Education* 19 July 1997: B1.
19 Gunsalus CK. Institutional structure to ensure research integrity. *Academic Medicine* 1993;**68**(9):(Suppl.).
20 Gunsalus CK. Preventing the need for whistleblowing: practical advice for university administrators. *Science and Engineering Ethics* (Opragen) 1998;**4**:51–64.
21 Gunsalus CK. How to blow the whistle and still have a career afterwards. *Science and Engineering Ethics* (Opragen) 1998;**4**:75–94.
22 Selsky A. *Houston Chronicle* Saturday 1 March 1997.

3: Pay cheques on a Saturday night: the changing politics and bureaucracy of research integrity in the United States

MARCEL C LA FOLLETTE

When viewed from the 21st century, the political bargain struck between the scientific community and the US government during the 1940s can perhaps seem idealistic and remote from modern-day policy concerns. Flushed with the success of their war work, scientists lobbied for the establishment of a semi-autonomous, decentralised system that would assure steady funding of basic and applied research through expansion of existing agencies and establishment of new ones.[1-3] In return, they optimistically promised discoveries and innovations that would fill "millions of pay envelopes on a peacetime Saturday night".[4]

Underpinning the scheme was the political assumption that scientists would be trustworthy stewards of public money. They would play an active role in allocating funds and guiding research agendas, and would retain institutional level autonomy over management and conduct of projects. Allowing scientists, in effect, to "self-regulate" their own activities seemed a reasonable approach at the time. Faith in science was high; the image of scientists, positive. Americans probably thought that if you can't trust a scientist (in their minds undoubtedly imagining Albert Einstein or Marie Curie), then who *can* you trust?

With such an arrangement, American taxpayers expected to reap considerable profit from the investment, even if some basic research proved irrelevant or unnecessary. Peace would be maintained; the economy would prosper. As progress rolled out of the laboratories in unending waves, the promise seemed fulfilled.

This fundamental expectation of integrity – rooted firmly in bureaucratic mechanisms to certify accountability – explains in part why scientific misconduct later became such a controversial political issue in the US. As Mark Frankel observes, scientists' professional autonomy is "not a right, but a privilege granted by society";[5] it is negotiated on the assumption that scientists will monitor their colleagues' performance.[6] The discovery, in the 1970s and 1980s, of faked and fabricated research in a few prestigious American institutions was disturbing enough to the politicians charged with oversight of the federal research system. When prominent scientists then reacted defensively to legislators' inquiries and even argued that the US Congress should "back off", lest scientific freedom be endangered, politicians, journalists, and the public reacted with dismay and disappointment. The subsequent years of squabbling over whether the "problem" consisted of only a "few bad apples" or a thoroughly "rotten barrel", as well as scientists' open questioning of federal authority to investigate allegations of fraud, furthered the erroneous impression that scientists in general cared little about integrity and only about preserving their autonomy.

How did the situation in the US shift from an atmosphere of such optimism and trust in the 1940s to today's increasing expansion of government regulation of research? How did a professional climate evolve in which accusations of unethical conduct can now trigger not just formal investigations and ruined careers but also years of litigation? This essay examines the particular circumstances and history of the controversy in the US, especially with regard to the biomedical sciences, and with attention to the lessons contained therein.

Erosion of trust

Acts of faked or misrepresented scientific and technical data, falsified professional credentials, misidentification of authorship, and plagiarism are neither contemporary inventions, nor limited to any one research field or national research system.[7–12] When problems have been uncovered, scientists around the world tend to act much the same: they characterise the offender as "aberrant", the episode as isolated, and the behaviour as probably prompted by stress, bad judgment, moral corruption, or all three. Only a few of the most notorious and sensational episodes before the 1970s are well-documented (such as the Piltdown skull forgery);[8,12] many allegations "survive" primarily in participants' memories or in the gossip of particular science departments. We have all listened to such stories handed around with the after-dinner coffee.

Until the 1980s, these tales remained largely within the family, receiving only intermittent attention from journalists. Even the first instance of fabricated data to receive significant public attention in the US, the William T Summerlin case, simmered only briefly in the headlines.[13] In 1974, Summerlin was working on skin cancer at the Sloan–Kettering Cancer Center in New York, investigating the use of tissue culture to facilitate genetically incompatible skin transplants. Before a meeting with the Center's director, Summerlin apparently darkened grafts on two white

33

mice to imply greater success in his experiments than they warranted. When confronted about his actions, Summerlin claimed that "mental and physical exhaustion", institutional pressure "to publicize the research", and "an unbearable clinical and experimental load" had "numbed" his judgment.[13] An investigating committee later concluded that he had lied about his research progress and fabricated supporting evidence, and eventually dismissed him from staff, but not without praising his "personal qualities of warmth and enthusiasm".[13]

This episode of the "painted mouse" contained several aspects common to subsequent high-profile cases: research with immediate salience to the audience; a popular scientist and/or powerful supporters; claims of momentary misjudgment or unusual stress; and an ambiguous resolution. Accused scientists sometimes maintained their jobs (and salaries) for years while institutional investigations dragged on; and the penalties, even for those proven to have committed fraud, were linked to loss of status (for example, directorships of laboratories or potential for tenure) and ability to participate in the life of science (for example, service on committees), rather than to substantial monetary fines, imprisonment, or loss of credentials.

As with most social and political change in the American democracy, media attention eventually served as the spotlight, drawing politicians like moths to a flame. The case that stimulated much of this increased publicity involved John Darsee, an up-and-coming researcher with prestigious mentors and affiliations (Emory University, Brigham and Women's Hospital in Boston, and Harvard Medical School).[14] The nature of the research involved (a multi-investigator, multi-institutional cardiology study funded by the National Institutes of Health [NIH]) helped to make the episode front page news in 1981, and although the primary allegations focused on data fabrication, the case also introduced a new cause for concern. Darsee had listed co-authors on many of his published articles, some of whom had not participated directly in the research described and were therefore given "honorary co-authorship". This practice had become standard in many laboratories, and none of the co-authors had objected when the articles were published, although most disavowed responsibility for the content after questions were raised. Two gadflies, biologists Ned Feder and Walter Stewart, used the Darsee case to draw attention to the ethics of authorship and to the editorial policies of scientific journals.[15] The case emphasised that each breach of integrity could have a negative impact on dozens, possibly hundreds, of other researchers. In the next phase of the controversy, it became clear that high-profile cases might even influence the public reputation of science overall.

Congress turns the spotlight on science

As delays in the university and government investigations of the Darsee case drew allegations of a cover-up, the resulting publicity stimulated congressional interest.[16] This phase represented action within what

Bruce LR Smith calls the third sphere of the accountability of science.[17] Scientists are initially accountable to their colleagues, operating according to the internally-generated norms that underpin the system of self-governance. Superimposed on this, Smith points out, is a level of "professionalized management" and "formal administrative structures", usually as part of universities; and then, finally, a "layer of public accountability". In the US prior to the 1980s, this third layer included laws and regulations relating to fiscal accountability, treatment of human subjects and animals, environmental quality, or national security, but not specifically to the personal integrity of researchers.[18]

The first formal congressional attention to scientific misconduct took place in two hearings on 31 March and 1 April 1981.[19] Albert Gore, then chairman of a subcommittee of the House of Representatives' Committee on Science and Technology, opened the hearing by stating, "We need to discover whether recent incidents are merely episodes that will drift into the history of science as footnotes, or whether we are creating situations and incentives in the biomedical sciences, and in all of 'Big Science', that make such cases as these 'the tip of the iceberg'."[19] "At the base of our investment in research", he continued, "lies the trust of the American people and the integrity of the scientific enterprise."[19]

A legislative hearing may seem a strange format in which to address topics like "trust" and "integrity" but it is actually well-suited to such discussions – especially when "no law has been violated", but there has been "an apparent betrayal of public trust".[20] As one political scientist explains, "By focusing on ethics rather than legality", legislative inquiries can help to crystallise political opinion about expected performance or acceptable goals and stimulate bureaucratic or institutional change.[20]

Chairs of legislative committees like Gore's, which are charged with authorisation (essentially the determination of an agency's overall mission and programmes) or oversight (monitoring an agency's fulfilment of that mission), wield power through press attention and political pressure. In the US, the process of "legislative oversight" (as opposed to passing laws or appropriating money) has grown alongside an expanding Presidency and federal bureaucracy.[21] As science and technology agencies like the National Science Foundation and NIH had grown throughout the 1960s and 1970s, the congressional scrutiny had kept pace.

The senior government officials who testified in the 1981 hearing seemed often oblivious to the legislators' concerns. Philip Handler, President of the National Academy of Sciences, called the issue "grossly exaggerated"; officials from the NIH echoed this assessment and denied the existence of widespread fraud in biomedical research.[19] When legislators expressed surprise that the agency had continued to fund scientists accused of wrongdoing – and even some who had been found guilty – the bureaucrats (a few of whom were scientists themselves) explained that the policy avoided "blacklisting" researchers who might be acquitted, even though it temporarily rewarded those later proven guilty.[19] As the hearing progressed, members of Congress angrily criticised this policy, warning that there is *no* political "entitlement" to uninterrupted federal funding, even for the most worthy scientist.[19]

Scientific fraud was still far from being a substantial political controversy, however. In 1981, Congress simply urged the scientific agencies and their grantees to investigate and resolve allegations swiftly and fairly, and to prevent future occurrences. Unfortunately, many in the mainstream scientific community greeted congressional interest as unreasonable, unwarranted, and restrictive of scientific freedom. The legislators, of course, knew that they had both a right and a responsibility to oversee federal activities and that their questions had been consistent with that role.

Complicating any political inquiry was the historic fragmentation of scientific research throughout the federal government, a situation mirrored on Capitol Hill. The House of Representatives committee that conducted the 1981 hearing had been assigned responsibility for reviewing laws, programmes, and government activities dealing with or involving *non-military* research and development; but a different House committee, chaired from the 1980s until 1995 by Democrat John Dingell of Michigan, oversaw the Department of Health and Human Services (and therefore the NIH). In the Senate, attention to science was similarly dispersed among several committees. Because even today no single committee has jurisdiction over all of science, no congressional hearing can presume to look at the issue of "scientific misconduct" in its entirety, only at those cases or issues related to the committee's jurisdiction. Instead, Congress, like the agencies who fund the research, has tended to approach the issue piecemeal, even though it clearly affects all parts of the research system.

Did John Dingell create the controversy?

The publicity given to John Dingell has prompted some to portray him as a villain who singlehandedly created this political controversy, probably dislikes scientists, and does not favour federal support for science. Yet, during most of his legislative career, Representative Dingell has fought tirelessly against fraud, waste, and abuse in all government-contracting activities. If federal funds are misspent, then scientists and their university employers look no different to him than dishonest defence contractors or bank executives. In fact, like most members of Congress, Dingell is intensely supportive of the scientific enterprise, working to increase research funding for his region and for particular topics.[22]

In April 1988, however, the politicians' disappointment was growing with every new instance of unethical conduct. On 11 April, scientists who had "blown the whistle" on fraudulent research described to a sub-committee of the House Committee on Government Operations how they had been vilified by colleagues and senior administrators and how the investigations prompted by their allegations had been repeatedly delayed at all levels.[23] The next day, at a hearing of another congressional committee, this time chaired by John Dingell, two young biologists, Margot O'Toole and Charles Maplethorpe, testified about how they had questioned research conducted in the MIT laboratory of Thereza Imanishi-Kari and published in an article in *Cell*.[24] Because one of the paper's co-authors was Nobel Laureate David Baltimore, journalists exploited the news that both Imanishi-Kari and Baltimore had dismissed O'Toole's initial queries about the data and discouraged her from raising questions formally or publicly. The "Baltimore case" (as it came to be known, although the specific accusations of misconduct were lodged against Imanishi-Kari not Baltimore) showed that even famous, well-regarded scientists could not avoid intense congressional scrutiny.[25,26] Maplethorpe testified that: "I felt that if I pursued the case at MIT and nothing happened then I would be the one to suffer."[24] Such statements naturally led journalists to speculate about potential cover-ups.

At the end of the hearing, Dingell gave notice that congressional inquiries would continue: "We are going to be visiting again about these matters," he promised.[27] Within days, quite by coincidence, another sensational episode became public. On 15 April 1988, psychologist Stephen J Breuning was indicted in federal court and charged with falsifying research project reports to the National Institute of Mental Health.[28–30] Scientists could no longer credibly argue – as they had at the 1981 hearing – that fraud was "not a problem".

Each of these various cases provided a different lesson. The Breuning case, for example, demonstrated that science did not always "self-correct", as scientists had insisted in their earlier attempts to forestall regulation. Breuning's research data had been widely reported and widely used: from 1980–1983, his published papers represented at least one-third of all scientific articles on the topic; citation analysis has since shown that, from 1981 to 1985, his work had "meaningful" impact on the field.[31] The research had also influenced treatment plans for hundreds of children. Fraudulent science could thus be unknowingly incorporated into practice just as it persisted undetected in the literature. Such examples shattered the illusion that either the scientific community or the universities had the problem under control.

The scientific community responds

In retrospect, it seems clear that scientific associations and universities could have moved more aggressively to re-articulate and publicise the basic norms of honesty and integrity that guide scientists' work, and to declare that unethical behaviour would not be tolerated or ignored. Instead, there was a tendency to blame the messengers or critics, and to perceive any questioning as an assault on the autonomy of government-funded scientific research. Unapologetic resistance to congressional suggestions of reform persisted for several years, especially in the biomedical research community. A *New England Journal of Medicine* (June 1988) editorial argued against establishment of *any* federal ethics oversight system and asserted that Congress was simply "responding to false impressions" and should therefore back off: "The biomedical-research community is willing and able to police itself and is taking steps to do so more effectively... Let us hope that Congress will give this process time to work."[32] The following year, the House Committee on Science and Technology heard more testimony from representatives of NIH, National Science Foundation, and various universities; they also questioned journal editors about the peer review process and the integrity of the published literature.[33] Chairman Robert A Roe, an ardent supporter of the federal research effort, stated bluntly that "scientific misconduct is a general problem that threatens the health of the scientific enterprise at all levels", and he appealed to scientists to act: "There will be no greater force for maintaining the integrity of scientific research than the science community itself... The federal government cannot fund science at ever greater levels and then turn its back on the problem of scientific misconduct."[33]

The efforts of some institutions and professional associations to develop guidelines or ethics codes were notable, such as those of the Association of American Medical Colleges and the Association of American Universities, as well as the work of groups like the American Psychological Association and the American Association for the Advancement of Science to promote integrity discussions through workshops, conferences, and other projects.[34,35] However, too many universities and organisations continued with business as usual. Scientific journals refused to withdraw tainted articles even after fraud was proven, fearful of being sued if even one co-author objected (see, for example, the fate of the co-authored articles of Robert Slutsky).[36–38] After Stephen E Breuning was indicted and pleaded guilty, more than fifty of his articles remained in dispute for months – Breuning refusing to discuss the matter publicly and the journals refusing to retract unless all authors agreed.[39]

The implications of these and similar episodes also reverberated within scientific publishing, reshaping journal review practices that had once relied solely on trust.[7] Scientific publishers and editors began to redefine their standards and expectations for how authors, reviewers, and editors should behave, and to articulate more formally the limits of their responsibilities, both legal and moral.

By the 1990s, political attention had turned away from the malefactors (perhaps because fewer of the accused were well-known scientists) and toward the quality of misconduct investigations.[40,41] NIH management practices were scrutinised and the ethics office eventually reorganised at congressional request.[42] Meanwhile, scientists continued to debate the limits of what should or should not be labelled as "misconduct",[43,44] and John Dingell expressed hope that the research community would eventually begin to "police itself".[40]

Whistleblowers

One of the most difficult policy issues that arose during this time involved the protection of those entangled in misconduct cases. There was evidence that some whistleblowers, especially if they were students or young scientists, had been ostracised, threatened, or otherwise retaliated against.[45] Scientists who were the targets of malicious or unfounded allegations themselves became victims of the political pressure to investigate. Every case seemed to attract unpleasant publicity, and a finding of innocence sometimes came too late to salvage a professional reputation. Those who wrote about or analysed misconduct also became the targets of vilification, drawing attacks simply for writing academic analyses or speaking out on ethical issues.

The concern for whistleblowers owes much to the tribulations of a single postdoctoral researcher, Margot O'Toole. When O'Toole repeatedly questioned data presented in an article co-authored by, among others, Thereza Imanishi-Kari and David Baltimore, she was warned that her scepticism would be harmful to her career.[25,46] Years later, an NIH investigation showed her questions to have been reasonable, O'Toole was praised as a hero, and *The New York Times* lauded her strength of character.[47] In the interval, however, her career had been damaged and, for many years, she was unable to find work as a scientist, while opponents caustically questioned her scientific competence and accused her of prolonging the dispute out of vindictiveness.[48,49]

To his credit, David Baltimore eventually apologised to O'Toole, and conceded that Congress indeed had the responsibility to oversee and investigate federally funded research.[50] He acknowledged that he had failed to treat a junior colleague's well-meant questions with appropriate respect, and later observed that, "This entire episode has reminded me of the importance of humility in the face of scientific data."[51] As a result of the controversy surrounding O'Toole, protections for whistleblowers received important attention early in the development of regulations.

Regulations cannot, however, reconstruct ruined careers. "Whistleblowers in American society have not fared well even when their allegations have eventually been substantiated," Mark Frankel notes.[5] Studies by the Office of Research Integrity have shown that the majority of whistleblowers experience some negative consequences, and many observers have argued that whistleblowers should therefore be allowed to make allegations anonymously. The close relationships within laboratories and departments can make it uncomfortable even to raise questions in good faith. One study found that while 30% of senior biochemists who "personally knew of severe incidents of misconduct" had taken no action, the majority had indeed acted, in ways ranging from direct confrontation to formal administrative report; however, the biochemists also indicated that they weighed any such action against the potential for harm to their own careers and potential embarrassment to the accused.[6] Yet, because federal regulations now require that every credible allegation be investigated, and a cry of "scientific misconduct" is an effective tool with which to punish a rival, enemy, or former employer, many scientists argue that all accusers should be forced to place their complaints and names on the record. If you instigate an inquiry, then you should be willing to be held accountable.

The quandary for universities and federal agencies has been to develop procedures that balance such views and protect the rights of *both* the accused and the accuser. If hearings and investigations are completely open and on the record, will that leave whistleblowers vulnerable to retaliation? If the process is closed and confidential, then does that inordinately increase the power of malicious or misguided accusations? One solution adapted by the NIH ethics office has been to offer limited anonymity, although few complaints have remained anonymous beyond the first contact, and even fewer of those have been substantive enough to warrant formal investigation.[52]

Whilst retaliation against a whistleblower who makes a report in good faith is now itself cause for inquiry by the National Science Foundation, and is condemned by many of the ethics guidelines published by professional societies, the biomedical agencies continue to maintain that retaliatory action, whilst wrong, should not be considered "scientific misconduct", leaving it to the institutions to investigate and punish according to their own rules. This issue, then, continues to attract debate and controversy, as all parties search for policies and procedures that will be fair, just, and effective.

The bureaucratic response

In addition to its high-profile hearings and excess of publicity, the "Baltimore case" had another significant impact on the course of events, in that it attracted considerable publicity to the quality of government misconduct investigations. In late 1994, the Office of Research Integrity issued a finding of misconduct against Imanishi-Kari, which she then appealed against.[53] In June 1996, the Departmental Appeals Board for the US Department of Health and Human Services ruled that the Office of Research Integrity had not proved either fabrication or falsification, and rejected the evidence on which the case had rested, so the case was officially closed over seven years after it had begun.

The National Science Foundation and National Institutes of Health, the two parts of the United States government most directly concerned with funding basic research, have responded quite differently to Congressional pressure to investigate misconduct. During the 1970s, concern about government ethics and contracting practices had resulted in the creation of special oversight offices throughout the Executive Branch. The head of each office, called an Inspector General, was assigned separate audit responsibility and charged with investigating any potential financial mismanagement or non-performance of duties by agency employees, grantees, and contractors. By placing its research misconduct unit within its Inspector General's office, the National Science Foundation avoided the stigma associated with a separate "ethics police force", and made a strong statement about the link between ethical behaviour and overall accountability for expenditure of federal funds. Since publishing its regulations in 1987, the Foundation has steadily refined its processes and mounted a number of major investigations without attracting significant congressional criticism.

At NIH, however, continued media scrutiny of new cases – and the agency's delays in investigating old ones – contributed to an atmosphere of bureaucratic confusion. Although NIH had begun to formulate its policies for grantees in 1981, Congress directed the Secretary of Health and Human Services in 1985 to develop regulations for all *applicants* for grants, contracts, and cooperative agreements, requiring them to report allegations and investigations to the government (Public Law 99-158), a requirement further strengthened with passage of additional legislation in 1993 (Public Law 103-43). An Office of *Scientific* Integrity was established for NIH, but both the office and the proposed guidelines attracted so much criticism from the biomedical community and the Congress that control of ethics investigations was eventually moved from NIH to its parent agency, the Public Health Service, within the Department of Health and Human Services, and the office renamed. The new Office of *Research* Integrity achieved somewhat more bureaucratic stability; but in Spring 2000, it was further reorganised. Responsibility for formal investigations was assigned elsewhere and the office's mandate changed to reflect increased federal involvement in ethical training for researchers.[54] At present, cases that require official inquiry are referred to the Department of Health and Human Services' Office of Inspector General, which is staffed primarily by attorneys and trained investigators.

The other recent attempt to bring consistency to federal policies is an effort to write a government-wide definition of misconduct. This effort, guided by the Office of Science and Technology within the White House, has been repeatedly delayed by bureaucratic and partisan politics, but regulations were finally published in December 2000 (see page 24) but will not be fully implemented for years. The progress (or lack of progress) in developing a consensus definition exemplifies how, in the US, admirable ideals and a desire to achieve worthy goals can become easily entangled in the bureaucratic processes of a lively democracy.

Authorship and plagiarism

One issue that government agencies did not initially anticipate was that of authorship, including plagiarism and disputes over credit. Although the Darsee case focused attention on authorship practices in journals (for example, who should or should not be listed as a co-author), this issue was generally considered to fall outside federal jurisdiction. Plagiarism – the deceptive presentation of another's text or ideas as one's own[55] – also seemed a peripheral concern, until government ethics investigators began to notice a significant number of complaints raised about plagiarism from (and in) grant proposals. Of the 75 allegations received by the National Science Foundation from 1 January 1989 to 31 March 1991, 40 dealt with plagiarism or other misappropriation of intellectual property.[56] Between

41

1993 and 1997, only 5% of the 150 investigations completed by the Office of Research Integrity involved plagiarism, but authorship disputes have now increased in the biomedical sciences as well.[57]

The consequent discussions about responsible authorship and co-authorship have helped to emphasise how complex those roles have become in modern science. Disputes involving co-authors have been exacerbated by the dramatic rise in collaborative research projects and the number of co-authors per publication in all fields.[58] By the mid-1990s, the Institute for Scientific Information was routinely describing hundreds of journal articles that listed over 100 authors apiece. The pressure to add more collaborators to a project – and hence to its publications – shows no indication of diminishing. To what extent has the value of authorship been eroded by these practices, and if the biomedical community cannot reverse the trend, then what rights and responsibilities should be assigned in the future to all partners in print?

Electronic publication – either through traditional journals or Internet circulation by individual authors – has changed the playing field dramatically. A computer can make plagiarism and alteration of photographic evidence relatively easy. Maintaining confidentiality and privacy, tracking errors in databases, and retrieving the effects of deliberate fraud and deception in data production and interpretation also defeat ordinary means of detection when there is no paper trail to follow, but only bits and bytes. Speed, in the new cyberlaboratory of global information networks, frequently outstrips wisdom and prudence. Monitoring electronic communications to guard against unethical practices involves an invasion of the private space of scientists, which seems initially unthinkable and yet may be one of the routes next proposed.

Prevention, especially through ethical mentoring of young scientists, thus takes on added importance. The development by scientific associations of clear standards and guidelines for conduct in the particular circumstances of their fields is an essential part of the process. In each research field, we will need to define new sets of scientific virtues that suit new times and new means of communication, but the transition period to the new era promises to be challenging for all stakeholders.

Insufficient data

Development of wise policies for prevention, investigation, and resolution of scientific misconduct cases continues to be hampered by insufficient data about the motivations, demographics, and extent of fraud. As the Editor of *Science*, Donald Kennedy, wrote following an episode involving his journal: "We need to know more about what motivates scientific misconduct and what can prevent against it," and especially what "disincentives" might prove effective in preventing it.[59]

What we *don't* know far outweighs what we *do* know.[60] One of the persistent questions of the 1980s was, "How much misconduct is there?"

Through 1999, the Office of Research Integrity was issuing a finding of misconduct in about one-third of the cases investigated, but this number (still only several hundred since the 1980s) reflects only those cases that had wound their way through various departmental and institutional reviews. After examining much of the available government statistics on misconduct cases, Edward Hackett has concluded that, "It is difficult to know if there is much or little misconduct in science, if the rate has risen or remained constant, or if variation in the number of reported cases indicates changes" in any of the relevant parameters.[61] It is safe to say, then, that whilst misconduct appears to be an aberration, and by no means reflective of an eroded integrity of science overall, the answer to the question asked in almost every forum on the topic since the 1980s remains unanswerable.

Information about who commits misconduct is equally sketchy. Most of the wrongdoers have been bright, accomplished scientists, who have engaged sometimes in honest and, other times, in dishonest research, that is, they have *chosen* to cheat. Many were rising rapidly in their careers, and had astonishing rates of production (but, then, so do many successful and honest scientists). No obvious link appears to exist between a predilection for unethical behaviour and any particular type of training or institutional employer, although the greater proportion of biomedical investigations in the US have, perhaps predictably, involved medical schools, where much of such government-funded research is conducted.[57] Although initially there were far fewer women than men accused of research fraud, this "gender gap", too, has begun to close.[57]

In all instances, the accused person has wilfully sacrificed personal and professional integrity to a vision of "science (or fame) at any cost". Many younger fraudsters exploited lax supervision to advantage. Few seemed fearful that conventional oversight or peer review would detect their deception or, even if it did, that there would be serious recrimination. Perhaps those scientists who fake experiments are risktakers, regarding the process as a game, as a way to outwit their peers, much like the art forger who believed that "only the experts are worth fooling, and the greater the expert, the greater the satisfaction of deceiving him."[62] As psychologists and sociologists explore such issues, we may eventually know the truth about "who" and "why" as well as how to deter problems in the future.

The dance of democracy

Does the American experience reflect flaws in the country's training, supervision, or values, or is this story reflective more of universal human and institutional failures? Now that the topic has been scrutinised for several decades and the list of documented and proven cases reaches into the hundreds, we might reasonably conclude that the urge to cheat seems to be an all-too-human feeling, and the tendency of scientific and academic institutions to prefer to ignore, dismiss, or cover up embarrassing ethical lapses to be (unfortunately) an international problem.

43

What does seem to be different is how each national research system or government reacts to allegations of fraud. The US scientific agencies, their bureaucratic heads, and Congress engaged for many years in a contentious, strident, and antagonistic battle characteristic of the "dance of democracy": a search for accountability within a complex system un-manageable by normal bureaucratic means. When the scientific community assured Americans that intellectual integrity and political accountability could be maintained through rigorous internal assessment ("peer review"), even in a rapidly expanding research system, they bound themselves to a delicate political bargain. Development of a sense of "entitlement" among the research community, and a lapsed sense of individual accountability, distorted this relationship and contributed to "moral amnesia" on the part of some of the leaders in American science. Congress, of course, always understood the bottom line: budgets change, priorities shift. The well-funded department of today may be pragmatically eliminated in a reorganisation tomorrow. Keeping the bargain was essential for maintaining the status quo.

Conclusion

Americans have been predisposed to like scientists and think well of them; but the original social contract was not a product of naivety. As Don K Price wrote, "Ever since Benjamin Franklin and Thomas Jefferson, Americans have been inclined to put their faith in a combination of democracy and science as a sure formula for human progress."[63] The economic linkage between basic research and the promised return on the federal investment gave society the upper hand; society could always withhold funding and call the scientists to accountability. The linkage also facilitated creation of a regulatory framework for scientific research, which did not exist before 1945, except for research directly related to military defence. Concern about potential abuse of human subjects and animals prompted expensive requirements for how (and whether) some research could be conducted; concern about environmental pollution began to restrict disposal of the chemical and biological byproducts of research.[18] Requiring universities to establish procedures and offices for investigating potential misconduct fitted this overall pattern and added to the regulatory burden.

Today, "leaving it to the scientists" or relying on "personal ideals and social controls" alone is no longer considered appropriate or prudent.[64] American scientists may be able to rebuild public and political trust in their integrity through future reliable performance; but the opportunity to forestall regulation is past. "Instead of a handshake giving generous funding along with broad discretion," Bruce Smith observes, "the pact between science and society will increasingly resemble a government contract, with much haggling over the fine print."[17] Combined with less discretionary funding available for basic research and increased public wariness of science, a return to those golden days of an *unblemished* reputation now seems only a dream for a lonely Saturday night.

References

1 Hart DM. *Forged consensus: science, technology, and economic policy in the United States, 1921–1953*. Princeton, NJ: Princeton University Press, 1998.

2 Kleinman DL. *Politics on the endless frontier: postwar research policy in the United States*. Durham, NC: Duke University Press, 1995.

3 Smith BLR. *American science policy since World War II*. Washington, DC: Brookings Institution, 1990.

4 Bush V. *Science – The endless frontier, a report to the president on a program for postwar scientific research*. Washington, DC: US Government Printing Office, 1945, 10.

5 Frankel MS. Scientific societies as sentinels of responsible research conduct. *Proc Soc Exp Biol* 2000;**224**:216, 218.

6 Braxton JM, Bayer AE. Personal experience of research misconduct and the response of individual academic scientists. *Science Technol Human Values* 1996;**21**:200, 206.

7 LaFollette MC. *Stealing into print: fraud, plagiarism, and other misconduct in scientific publishing*. Berkeley, CA: University of California Press, 1992.

8 Weiner JS. *The Piltdown forgery*. New York: Oxford University Press, 1955.

9 Rieth A. *Archaeological fakes*. Translated by D Imber. New York: Praeger Publishers, 1970.

10 Broad WJ, Wade N. *Betrayers of the truth: fraud and deceit in the halls of science*. New York: Simon and Schuster, 1982.

11 Kohn A. *False prophets: fraud and error in science and medicine*. New York: Basil Blackwell, 1986.

12 Spencer F. *Piltdown: a scientific forgery*. New York: Oxford University Press, 1990.

13 Hixson J. *The patchwork mouse*. Garden City, NJ: Anchor Press/Doubleday, 1976.

14 Relman AS. Lessons from the Darsee affair. *N Engl J Med* 1983;**308**:1415–17.

15 Stewart WW, Feder N. The integrity of the scientific literature. *Nature* 1987;**325**:207–14.

16 LaFollette MC. A foundation of trust: scientific misconduct: congressional oversight, and the regulatory response. In: Braxton JM, ed. *Perspectives on scholarly misconduct in the sciences*. Columbus, OH: Ohio State University Press, 1999, pp.11–41.

17 Smith BLR. The accountability of science. *Minerva* 1996;**34**:47–8, 54.

18 US Congress. House. *The regulatory environment for science, science policy study background*. Report no. 10 to the Committee on Science and Technology. 99th Congress, 2nd session. Washington, DC: US Government Printing Office, 1986.

19 US Congress. House. *Fraud in biomedical research, hearings before the Committee on Science and Technology, Subcommittee on Investigations and Oversight*. 97th Congress, 1st session. Washington, DC: US Government Printing Office, 1981.

20 Griffith ES. *Congress: its contemporary role*, 3rd edn. New York: New York University Press, 1961.

21 Aberbach JD. *Keeping a watchful eye: the politics of congressional oversight*. Washington, DC: Brookings Institution, 1990, p. 22.

22 Savage JD. *Funding science in America: Congress, universities, and the politics of the academic pork barrel*. Cambridge: Cambridge University Press, 1999.

23 US Congress. House. *Scientific fraud and misconduct and the federal response*. Hearing of the Committee on Government Operations, Subcommittee on human resources and intergovernmental relations. 100th Congress, 1st session, 11 April 1988. Washington, DC: US Government Printing Office, 1988.

24 US Congress. House. *Scientific fraud and misconduct in the National Institutes of Health Biomedical Grant Programs*. Hearing of the Committee on Energy and Commerce, Subcommittee on Oversight and Investigations. 100th Congress, 1st session, 12 April 1988. Washington, DC: US Government Printing Office, 1988.

25 Sarasohn J. *Science on trial: the whistle blower, the accused, and the Nobel laureate*. New York: St Martin's Press, 1993.

26 Kevles DJ. *The Baltimore case: a trial of politics, science, and character*. New York: WW Norton, 1998.

27 Greenberg DS. Fraud inquiry: NIH on the capitol griddle (continued). *Science and Government Report* 1988;**18**(1 May):3–6.

28 Valentine PW. Drug therapy researcher is indicted. *The Washington Post* 16 April 1988;**111**:A1, A14.
29 Wheeler DL. Researcher is indicted for falsifying data and impeding investigation of his work. *Chronicle of Higher Education* 27 April 1988;**34**:A4, A12.
30 Zurer PS. Researcher criminally charged with fraud. *Chem Engineering News* 25 April 1988;**66**:5.
31 Garfield E. The impact of scientific fraud. In: *Guarding the guardians: research on peer review*. Proceedings of the 1st Internat Congr Peer Review in Biomedical Publication. Chicago, Illinois, 10–12 May 1989, p. 53.
32 Angell M, Relman AS. A time for congressional restraint. *N Engl J Med* 1988;**318**:1462–3.
33 US Congress. House. Committee on Science, Space, and Technology. *Maintaining the integrity of scientific research*. 101st Congress, 2nd session. Washington, DC: US Government Printing Office, 1990, pp. 3–4.
34 Johnson D. From denial to action: academic and scientific societies grapple with misconduct. In: Braxton JM, ed. *Perspectives on scholarly misconduct in the sciences*. Columbus, OH: Ohio State University Press, 1999, pp. 42–74.
35 Steneck NH. Research universities and scientific misconduct: history, policies, and the future. In: Braxton JM, ed. *Perspectives on scholarly misconduct in the sciences*. Columbus, OH: Ohio State University Press, 1999, pp. 75–98.
36 Engler RL, Covell JW, Friedman PJ, Kitcher PS, Peters RM. Misrepresentation and responsibility in medical research. *N Engl J Med* 1987;**317**:1383–9.
37 Friedman PJ. Research ethics, due process, and common sense. *JAMA* 1988;**260**:1937–8.
38 Dalton R. Journals slow to retract Slutsky research errors. *The Scientist* 1988; **2**(7 March):1,4.
39 Hostetler AJ. Fear of suits blocks retractions. *The Scientist* 1987;**1**(19 October):1–2.
40 US Congress. House. *Scientific fraud and misconduct: The institutional response*. Hearing of the Committee on Energy and Commerce, Subcommittee on Oversight and Investigations. 101st Congress, 1st session, 9 May 1989. Washington, DC: US Government Printing Office, 1989.
41 US Congress. House. *Scientific fraud*. Hearing of the Committee on Energy and Commerce, Subcommittee on Oversight and Investigations. 101st Congress, 2nd session, 14 May 1990. Washington, DC: US Government Printing Office, 1990.
42 Greenberg DS. Fraud inquiry: harsh treatment for NIH on Capitol Hill. *Science and Government Report* 1988;**18**(15 April):1.
43 Schachman HK. What is misconduct in science? *Science* 1993;**261**:148–9, 183.
44 Buzzelli DE. The definition of misconduct in science: a view from NSF. *Science* 1993;**259**:584–5, 647–8.
45 Kuznik F. Fraud busters. *The Washington Post Magazine* 1991;(14 April):22–6, 31–3.
46 Zurer PS. Whistleblower rejects apology by Baltimore. *Chem Engineering News* 1991; **69** (13 May):7.
47 Hilts PJ. Hero in exposing science hoax paid dearly. *New York Times* 1991; (22 March): A1, B6.
48 Culliton BJ. Baltimore cleared of all fraud charges. *Science* 1989;**243**:727.
49 Culliton BJ. Whose notes are they? *Science* 1989;**244**:765.
50 Zurer PS. Scientific whistleblower vindicated. *Chem Engineering News* 1991;**69**(8 April): 35–6,40.
51 Anonymous. David Baltimore's mea culpa. *Science* 1991;**252**:769–70.
52 Price AR. Anonymity and pseudonymity in whistleblowing to the US Office of Research Integrity. *Acad Med* 1998;**73**(May):467–72.
53 Anonymous. ORI finds misconduct against Dr Imanishi-Kari. *ORI Newsletter* 1994;**3**(1) (December):1.
54 Office of the Secretary, Office of Public Health and Science, US Department of Health and Human Services. Statement of organization, functions, and delegations of authority. *Federal Register* 2000;**65**(93)(12 May):30600–1.
55 LaFollette MC. Avoiding plagiarism: some thoughts on use, attribution, and acknowledgment. *J Inform Ethics* 1994;**3**(2):25–35.
56 Office of Inspector General. *Semiannual report to the Congress* Number 4 (1 October 1990– 31 March 1991). Washington, DC: National Science Foundation, 1991.
57 Office of Research Integrity. *1999 Annual Report*. Washington, DC: 2000.
58 McDonald KA. Too many co-authors? *Chronicle of Higher Education* 1995;**41**(28 April):A35–6.

59 Kennedy D. Reflections on a retraction. *Science* 2000;**289**:1137.
60 Anderson MS. Uncovering the covert: research on academic misconduct. In: Braxton JM, ed. *Perspectives on scholarly misconduct in the sciences*. Columbus, OH: Ohio State University Press, 1999, pp. 283–314.
61 Hackett EJ. A social control perspective on scientific misconduct. In: Braxton JM, ed. *Perspectives on scholarly misconduct in the sciences*. Columbus, OH: Ohio State University Press, 1999, pp. 101–2.
62 Hebborn E. *Drawn to trouble: confessions of a master forger*. New York: Random House, 1993, p. 218.
63 Price DK. *The scientific estate*. Cambridge, MA: The Belknap Press of Harvard University Press, 1965, p. 1.
64 Kassirer JP. The frustrations of scientific misconduct. *N Engl J Med* 1993;**328**:1634.

PART II
THE HISTORY OF FRAUD
AND MISCONDUCT

4: Research misconduct 1974–1990: an imperfect history

STEPHEN LOCK

Not one of the four working papers for the 1999 Edinburgh Consensus Conference[1] cited any reference before 1990. In part, this might reflect the difficulty of literature searches for earlier years; in part, constraints on the contribution's length and purpose; in part, the priorities in the documents to stress the importance of a subject neglected in many anciens regimés, and particularly in Britain. Yet surely such neglect also implied that nothing could be learnt from history – that times past could be ignored because little had happened. A similar neglect in the literature on research fraud has been geographical, with some authors failing to cite events in other parts of the world. A major and excellent book[2] on the Baltimore case, for example, fails to cite any development in Europe, whereas a simple literature search would have disclosed major cases of research fraud and farsighted initiatives in some countries.

Nevertheless, an emphasis on a rounded history of any subject is important, not merely in its own right but because it contains important lessons. To ignore others' contributions is to diminish a subject as well as the authors. The thoughtful books by Medawar (1979),[3] Broad and Wade (1982),[4] and Kohn (1986);[5] the comprehensive reports from the Association of American Medical Colleges (1982),[6] the Institute of Medicine (1982),[7] and the Association of American Universities (1988);[8] as well as the incisive articles by Majerus (1982),[9] Relman (1983),[10] and Maddox (1987),[11] all testify to the activity on the research fraud front before the 1990s, which had often anticipated the discussions as well as the solutions proposed "anew" at Edinburgh and other forums. In 1999 the British General Medical Council, for instance, made the ludicrous statement that, compared with the well-established pattern of research misconduct in the USA, it had not had "strong evidence of such a problem" in Britain.[12] A mere glance at the second edition of this book (1996) would have shown 14 instances in the public domain, many dealt with by the GMC itself, let alone the more anecdotal suggestions of other cases.

51

So history has as an important role in this subject as in many others (and ironically for this topic in at least one country – Denmark – its committee on scientific dishonesty would classify the failure to acknowledge previous contributions at the least as a transgression of scientific etiquette). This said, however, here I will restrict my account largely to the period from 1974 to 1990, and to examples from biomedicine. To be sure, there were earlier cases (discussed in major books on the subject,[3,4] and concern about the existence of fraud was voiced in eras and by people as diverse as 1664 with Robert Boyle (who cited "philosophicall robbery" [plagiarism] as a prime reason for creating the Royal Society's journal) and 1934 with Dorothy L Sayers (whose detective story *Gaudy Night* hinges on a case of fraud[13]). There are also other disciplines in which fraud has occurred: anthropology with Piltdown Man, for example (probably just a gentle hoax), or psychology (Sir Cyril Burt's much disputed work on intelligence quotients).

One immediate concern is when does journalism cease and history begin? Obviously nobody would be as draconian as Chairman Mao, who, when asked about the main effects of the French revolution, replied that it was too early to say. Most historians, however, would maintain that history cannot really begin until the important documents are in the public domain, often 30 years after the event. Even so, this objection has not stopped historians from writing the history of yesterday, with excellent accounts of the beginnings of HIV/AIDS, for example. So here I shall use the Swiss historian Jacob Burkhardt's definition of history: "What will interest future generations", taking 1974 as a watershed and continuing mostly only until 1990. The account will be imperfect. It is not comprehensive, nor indeed nearly as full as in the previous two editions of this book (although it will use several of the passages in it from my own and other articles). Instead I will use some of the classic cases to brush pivotal points into the perspective as it appears at the beginning of this new millennium. If this account seems unduly acerbic, it is because of my personal involvement with a seemingly unmovable scene for over 21 years.

Shock horror – start of the modern story: 1974 and Summerlin

The modern story really starts only in 1974 when, at the Sloan-Kettering institute in New York, William Summerlin faked transplantation results, darkening transplanted skin patches in white mice with a black felt-tip pen, and alleging that human corneas had been successfully transplanted into rabbits. Sir Peter Medawar, who was present at the latter demonstration, has given a good and amusing account of prevailing attitudes at the time, which led fellow scientists to keep quiet about results they just did not believe.[3] Admitting that he had been a moral coward at the time, Medawar said that he believed that the whole demonstration was either a confidence trick or a hoax. Though subsequently Summerlin's boss, the celebrated immunologist Robert Good, resigned from the directorship of the Institute, the general reaction wasn't the shock horror that research fraud was to evoke later: instead, there was a general feeling that Summerlin must have had a nervous breakdown through overwork, and he was sent away on a year's sick leave, and on full pay.

Only after the series of *anni horribili* – the year-by-year revelations of dishonest practices – did the US scientific community come to recognise that a small amount of fraud was a feature of scientific research. So, among others, we had Vijay Soman, a diabetologist who plagiarised parts of a paper sent to his boss for peer review; John Darsee a cardiologist with numerous papers and conference abstracts all based on invented results; Robert Slutsky, a radiologist, who at one time was publishing one paper every 10 days, many based on faked results. The circumstances were also unexpected: not only did all work in major centres – Soman at Yale, Darsee at Harvard, and Slutsky at the University of California, San Diego – but they also involved others, sometimes distinguished seniors, as co-authors of the fraudulent papers.

Such cases gave rise to soul-searching, official inquiries and recommendations (some described elsewhere in this book). However, before I shall describe the reactions, let us look again at 1975, the year in which the Summerlin case excited so much attention. To search carefully in the history of any topics is almost always to find an antecedent case to the classic "first" description. With HIV/AIDS, for example, we now know of instances well before the "official" first case of the airline steward in the 1980s. In Britain the fraudster reported in 1975 was probably forgotten because he was one of several cases of a variety of unprofessional behaviour coming before the GMC, reported only in the back pages of the *BMJ*. Nevertheless, the case of Dr Sedgwick[14] shared with subsequent cases what was subsequently to be seen, incorrectly, as a major feature of scientific fraud in Britain – falsification of data for a multicentre drug trial, involving a general practitioner taking part for the money. Unfortunately, this and the early later cases enabled the grandees of the British Establishment to inhibit future discussions by saying that any fraud involved only ill-qualified family doctors practising a poor standard of medicine and motivated by greed, and that fraud in academia did not occur.

An early UK case unrecognised: 1975 and JP Sedgwick

This family doctor from High Wycombe had agreed with a pharmaceutical company to coordinate and take part in a trial of an antihypertensive drug. He returned 101 completed clinical trial forms, many of which contained forged signatures of the seven other participating doctors, and results that showed that the active drug was having a uniform and consistent effect that was appreciably different from test results from other sources. Reported by the company to the GMC, Dr Sedgwick had his name removed from the Medical Register.

Three "classic" US cases: 1979 and Vijay Soman; 1981 and John Darsee; 1985 and Robert Slutsky

Vijay Soman

Soman was an assistant professor of medicine at the Yale School of Medicine, who plagiarised parts of a manuscript sent in 1978 by the *New England Journal of Medicine* for peer review to his boss, Philip Felig, who passed the job on to him. Subsequently Soman and Felig published an article on the same topic, insulin binding in anorexia nervosa, in the *American Journal of Medicine*. Accused of plagiarism and conflict of interest, Felig seemed to settle the difficulties by stating that the work had been completed before they had received the paper for review. But its author, Dr Helena Wachslicht-Rodbard, a young researcher at the National Institutes of Health (NIH), who during this episode was to switch to hospital practice, persisted with her complaints. An inquiry by Dr Jeffrey Flier, a Boston diabetologist, in February 1980 showed that these were justified. Not only had Soman copied her manuscript, but most of the data in his own joint study had been faked. A subsequent investigation soon after found that, of 14 articles, only two could be approved, and the data were either missing or fraudulent in the remaining 12 (10 of them with Felig as co-author). All these articles were retracted by Felig.

This case is important as it highlighted several themes that were to feature strongly in subsequent cases. Firstly, there was an abuse of editorial peer review. This was something that had often featured as anecdotal accusations by angry authors in the past but had rarely been documented (though it has occurred again since this episode). Secondly, there was the involvement of a distinguished figure as a "gift" author, who had put his name to work with which he had not been associated – indeed, he could not have been because the work had not been done and the results were invented. Thus the episode was a personal tragedy for Felig, who resigned from a prestigious post at Columbia University, to which he had been appointed while the episode was unfolding. Thirdly, in these early days the authorities did not know how to react. They were hesitant about instigating a full and proper inquiry into an accusation made against a senior figure, and only Wachslicht-Roadbard's persistence brought about the disclosures.

John Darsee

Darsee was a Harvard research worker in cardiology, who was seen to falsify data during a laboratory study. His overall head of department, the distinguished cardiologist Eugene Braunwald, decided that this was a single bizarre act and allowed him to continue to work under close supervision, but terminated his NIH fellowship. Six months later, however, it became clear that Darsee's data in a multicentre study of treatments to protect the ischaemic myocardium were different from those at the three other units taking part. Harvard Medical School set up a committee of investigation, as did the NIH and Emory University, where Darsee had also worked. It emerged that Darsee had committed an extensive series of frauds, originating in his undergraduate days at Notre Dame University and continuing at Emory and Harvard. These included non-existent patients or collaborators, and invented data, as in the multicentre trial. There were also procedures and results that on reflection were virtually impossible: drawing blood from the tail veins of 200 rats weekly for all of their 90-week lifespan, and obtaining venous blood specimens (including from a 2-year-old child). In all, during his career Darsee published over 100 papers and abstracts, many of them in prestigious journals and with distinguished co-authors; many of them had to be retracted.

Possibly until recently, more ink has been shed on Darsee's case than on any other. In part, this was because it was the first major publicised case that was not an isolated blemish on the face of science (not mad – rather, bad); in part, because it concerned prestigious institutions, co-authors, and journals; in part, because of the charismatic personality of one of the central figures; in part, because it started the whole debate about the rights and wrongs of authorship (particularly gift authorship), data retention, the supervision of juniors, and the management of suspected cases of fraud. There was also the realisation of the pressure to publish – and not merely important work but anything that showed a department's activity, though the results should somehow be positive. Finally, the case also shifted the whole climate of feeling of trust to thinking the unthinkable – the possibility that things might not be as they seemed. There was also the new concept: once a crook, often always a crook – Darsee was found to have had a long history of faking his results in different projects and in different settings.

All these ramifications are ably explored in Marcel LaFollette's book,[13] and also in her revised article in this volume (Chapter 3). A particularly cogent account of why Darsee was trusted in the conditions prevailing at the time was provided by his former mentor, Eugene Braunwald.[15] This episode also shows the inadequacy of editorial peer review for detecting fraud (although two workers at the NIH were subsequently to demonstrate some egregious errors in Darsee's papers[16]), as well as the role of attempts by other workers to replicate results in revealing its existence.

Unlike some other disciplines, such as chemistry or physics, a lack of replication is a feature of research in medicine, given that it is often complex and expensive, and there is little enthusiasm by peers for merely confirmatory work. Nevertheless, failure to replicate results has occasionally brought other medical research frauds to light, as in the case of Claudio Milanese, an Italian immunologist who had claimed that IL-4A, a lymphokine, induced interleukin-2 receptors.[17] Later research showed that IL-4A did not exist. Finally, subsequent research showed the depressing result that, although Darsee's articles had been retracted from the literature – and that this fact was reflected in the electronic databases – these were still being cited in the literature, not in articles on research fraud but as references in papers on the very topic with which Darsee's fraudulent research had allegedly been concerned.[18]

Robert Slutsky

Slutsky was a resident in cardiological radiology at the University of California, San Diego, who between 1978 and 1985 was the author or co-author of 137 articles. The possibility of fraud was raised by an astute referee who queried apparently identical statistical results for two separate sets of data in consecutive articles that he had to read when Slutsky applied for promotion.[19] An inquiry found experiments and measurements that had never been done, incorrect procedures, and reports of statistical analyses that had never been performed. A committee of investigation was set up and, after interviewing co-workers, looking at lab notebooks, and reading the articles, it classified these as valid (77 articles), questionable (49), or fraudulent (12). Some of these last were retracted, and a few statements of validity were also published.

This is yet another important case, illustrating several other features about research misconduct:

- There was Slutsky's high productivity: at one stage he was producing one paper every 10 days (and on diverse subjects), which occasioned little but admiration from his colleagues.
- Again, many of the latter were happy to accept gift authorship.
- There was the way in which this junior research worker had managed to escape any supervision of his research by his seniors. There was the inordinate amount of work involved for the committee of inquiry, which had to read the articles, look at the lab books, and consult the co-authors.
- Finally, there was the curious behaviour of several journals, which either declined to insert any retraction or statement of validation (sometimes but not always on legal grounds) or, if they did so, tended to do this in such terms as to make the retractions non-retrievable on electronic databases.[19]

All countries, all disciplines

In the subsequent discussions and reports (most of them in the weekly scientific and medical journals), two important facts emerged. Firstly, research fraud did affect all disciplines: articles appeared showing that Admiral Peary had not reached the pole, a German graduate student in chemistry had spiked the starting material in an experiment on enantio-selectivity, a professor at Chandigarh University claimed to have found fossils in the Himalayas that in reality had come from several other different parts of the world, while recently Karl Sabbagh has documented a scandal well known in botanical circles since the 1930s of a professor who transferred plants from Teesside to the Scottish island of Rum.[20] Secondly, it affected all countries, whether Western or the then Iron-Curtain ones, and sometimes cases from there brought out new points or emphasised old ones in a particularly dramatic manner. Such was the case in Australia, for, as Norman Swan pointed out in a striking paragraph in the second edition of this book,[21] in two instances there were the classic features of scientific fraud. Whistleblowers often come off worse than the fraudster; the checks and balances of fraud do not stop fraud; institutions care more about their reputations than the integrity of science, and, when powerful men are involved, their peers "turn into wimps who are prepared to use ad hominem arguments rather than objectivity".

Too perfect studies on the pill: 1981 and Michael Briggs

Michael Briggs was the foundation professor of endocrinology at Deakin University, Geelong, whose specialty was the biology and safety of oral contraceptives. A few years after his arrival, however, questions began to be raised about his research, in particular the high compliance and low dropout rates of his studies. These gained further impetus when hormone tests allegedly performed at the Alfred Hospital in Melbourne were found not to have been done, and nurses allegedly recruited for a study at Geelong had not been asked. When Dr Jim Rossiter, the chair of the university ethics committee, checked on Briggs's qualifications, he found that his PhD from Cornell did not exist.

Thereafter the management of this case became fraught with difficulties. The university chancellor refused Rossiter's request to obtain specialist advice and subsequently for a committee of inquiry to be set up, even though Briggs had failed to reply to a letter asking for a response to Rossiter's questions. Subsequently an inquiry, which had been established by the vice-chancellor, was quashed on an appeal by Briggs (supported by the university staff association) to the university visitor, who stated that it had been improperly created. Further moves were also stymied when Briggs resigned and constitutionally any inquiry had to stop.

Nevertheless, the whistleblowers, and particularly Rossiter, had been harassed by threatening phone calls in the middle of the night, while there was an atmosphere of unhappiness at the university, which was split between those who supported Briggs and those who did not. A subsequent official inquiry into the university's procedures explained some of the anomalies, although several of the participants found it evasive on some details and, as always, such painful episodes are hard to adjust to. The whole of Swan's extended account makes a fascinating read of how personalities can affect events so profoundly, but to me the particular emphasis to come out of it all is the credulity of scientists when faced with a charming conman, something also seen in the Darsee case. Geelong is a small town, and to anybody with a slightly sceptical frame of mind the numbers of women allegedly recruited for these studies are unbelievable (as Darsee's bleeding of the rats' tails should have been). So peer reviewers should be counselled to think the unthinkable.

A "Man of Australia" humbled: 1988 and William McBride

Among the first to describe the teratogenic effects of thalidomide on the human fetus, William McBride, a Sydney obstetrician, had been honoured by a national subscription enabling him to set up and direct a private research institute, Foundation 41. Here in 1982 a junior scientist, Phil Vardy, asked his boss about a large number of discrepancies between the details printed in a paper in the *Australian Journal of Biological Sciences* and those in the experiments on rabbits he had participated in.

These so-called results made hyoscine (an anticholinergic drug used in travel sickness preparations) seemingly a teratogen. A version of the paper was submitted in evidence in a court case in the USA, where McBride was appearing as an expert witness alleging that a related preparation, Debendox/Bendectin had caused fetal deformities. Given the costs of the defence, the drug was withdrawn from the market, although no suit was ever won.

Once he was certain that he was dealing with scientific fraud, Vardy confronted McBride, but got nowhere – eventually he and most of the other junior scientists at the foundation left for other jobs. Rather later, Norman Swan, a medically qualified journalist and broadcaster, met Vardy and was shown the drafts of the paper and the progressive changes in the data. Swan made a radio documentary, which was broadcast in December 1987 but, despite the furore, it was clear that the Australian scientific community lacked procedures for dealing with such accusations – especially since Foundation 41 was a private institution, with McBride as its head. It took six months before the calls for an independent inquiry were met. This, chaired by the former Chief Justice of Australia, Sir Henry Gibbs, found that McBride had indeed committed scientific fraud, whereupon he resigned, only to be reinstated after the foundation's board had been ousted. Eventually, after a prolonged hearing, which cost both sides millions of dollars, and where in 1991 McBride admitted to publishing false and misleading data, the Medical Tribunal of New South Wales found him guilty of scientific fraud. This was in February 1993 and it took the tribunal another five months to strike him off the Medical Register.

This case (which again is a condensed account from the highly instructive article by Norman Swan in the second edition of this book[21]), illustrates three main points:

- Even though cases of scientific fraud had been reported in other countries carrying out major research, and mechanisms devised to deal with them, Australia was still largely without proposed procedures.
- There was a particularly difficult problem where an institution's governance was in private hands and, moreover, where it was its director who was accused.
- Finally, it illustrates how far even distinguished workers are prepared to go to vindicate a thesis – something that Sir Peter Medawar called the

"Messianic complex" (which he regarded as the most important cause of fraud of the lot).[3]

Having become obsessed by the idea that many agents might be teratogenic and constitute an unrecognised hazard to the fetus, McBride went to extreme lengths to prove this. Indeed, in an earlier incident he had tried to implicate imipramine, a tricyclic antidepressant, as a teratogen, again without any evidence.

Reactions by the community

As is clear by now, each country reacted in its own particular way (echoing Tolstoy's opening phrase in *Anna Karenina*: "Each unhappy family is unhappy after its own fashion"). Once galvanised, the USA, where Congress became heavily involved with John Dingell as an incisive and aggressive chairman, set up a body for looking into accusations of fraud in research sponsored by the National Institutes of Health. It soon altered the direction of this when the founding organisation, the Office of Scientific Integrity (based on dialogue among peers), was shown to have failed, particularly by its denial of fairness ("due process") to the accused and whistleblower. Since its creation in June 1992, its successor, the Office of Research Integrity, is generally acknowledged to have worked well. It has published regular reports and has set up task forces to look into individual problems, including the definition of misconduct and problems encountered by whistleblowers. To be sure, it has had problems, and in two major instances those implicated were eventually exonerated, but most people agree that this merely reflects problems inherent in any legal process and is no reason for abandoning the policing of a probably small but important element in scientific deviance – certainly major cases continue to be reported from major centres with all the familiar features.

Other countries where the problem seems to have been addressed head-on are the Nordic bloc, where each nation has established a central committee working in a slightly different way. All these responses are detailed in the individual chapters in this book. Conversely, the anciens regimes – Britain, France, and Germany – have been much slower to tackle the problem. One common theme behind this seemed to be a feeling by the grandees that science does not wash its dirty linen in public: that such matters are best ignored or discussed privately and any conclusions brushed under the carpet. Thus in the first edition of this book (1993), two French commentators wrote: "As identification of fraud is not organised in France, and known cases remain confidential, no mechanism for dealing with it exists ... Mechanisms for dealing with fraud at the publication stage do not exist. Papers disclosing misconduct on fraud such as those published by French or American journals, seem unlikely to be published in France in the next decade."[22] In the second edition (1996) Stegemann-Boehl commented: "Before the introduction of specific misconduct provisions can be discussed in Germany, it must be generally accepted that misconduct in science is more than a sign of decadence in the New World, and that the prevailing strategy of muddling through must give way also in Germany to a discussion of the problem within the scientific community as well as by the public ... Very likely, the prestige of science will suffer more as a result of accidentally discovered scandals than as a result of a discussion which makes it clear that the problem has been recognised."[23]

An exception to the behaviour of the anciens regimes might seem to have been Britain, where, spurred by two of the editors of this book (Stephen Lock and Frank Wells), the Royal College of Physicians set up a committee in 1990, producing a report in the following year.[24] This leant heavily on earlier documents, in particular that produced by Harvard Medical School (substantive and later document),[25] reproducing both its guidelines and the statement on authorship by the International Committee of Medical Journal Editors as appendices, and recommending that all authorities should adopt a twofold approach: promoting high standards of research and developing a mechanism for the management of complaints of research fraud – publicising the name of the screener and setting up the threefold process of receipt, inquiry, and investigation.

There, however, matters stopped. The committee's suggestion that a central organisation, such as one of the Nordic central bodies or the US Office of Scientific Integrity, should be set up was dropped. Unusually the Royal College held no press conference to launch the report, as it does for virtually all of its reports. A few years later, when I asked the registrar to question the postgraduate deans about their experiences of implementing the report, virtually none of them knew that the report had charged them with this responsibility, and very few had even heard of the report. The whole situation was indeed very similar to an earlier episode where the British Establishment had shortchanged society by failing to admit that there had been lax standards in the ethics of some medical research procedures. Only the persistence of an outsider, Maurice Pappworth (who documented some egregiously unethical research), had resulted in belated action being taken to *recommend* the establishment of research ethics committees (and even today these are still not a statutory requirement).[26]

Nevertheless, as this new edition also shows, belatedly the anciens régimes have begun to take some action, even if this has still only been halfhearted and mostly talk. In each instance, action has arisen from a pivotal case, and here I will stray past my self-imposed limits to describe the case that at least led to the first conference on the subject in Britain, at Edinburgh in 1999 (well after two meetings had been held in Warsaw and one in Beijing, let alone many other nations).

Galvanising the British at last? 1995 and the Pearce affair

Although the formation of the Danish committee was done in the anticipation of some future instance, most countries have examined the problem in response to a particularly egregious case. In Britain, as I have stated, the feeling among the medical *Prominenten* was that research fraud was a squalid affair confined to poorly qualified and practising general practitioners, and hence could be dealt with through the disciplinary machinery of the General Medical Council. Thus, even though an early case in Britain did concern a consultant, any suggestion that this showed that fraud existed in hospital or academic practice could still be dismissed because the malefactor was an overseas-qualified psychiatrist whose motivation had been greed (see Chapter 5 for a discussion of Dr Siddiqui). It took another, and more high profile case before it became obvious that in Britain, just as elsewhere, fraud also affected research in hospitals and laboratories.

In 1995 Malcolm Pearce, a British gynaecologist, was removed from the Medical Register for fraud: he had published two papers in the *British Journal of Obstetrics and Gynaecology* describing work that had never taken place. In the first paper Pearce claimed that he had successfully relocated a 5-week-old ectopic embryo via the cervix; he had two co-authors, including the editor of the journal, who was also the then president of the Royal College of Obstetricians and Gynaecologists and Pearce's boss at St George's Hospital Medical School in London. The second fraudulent claim was of a complex trial in 191 women with the rare syndrome of polycystic ovary disease and recurrent abortion. After a meticulous inquiry, conducted by a knowledgeable and determined dean of the medical school on the lines recommended in the Royal College of Physicians report, Pearce was dismissed from his post and reported to the GMC, while both articles were retracted, as were subsequently several others at the request of the special investigative committee.

By now, even if some of the features of the Pearce case were new to those in Britain, regrettably it illustrated yet again some of the lessons learnt elsewhere. As well as the demonstration that academics could commit research fraud, there was also the question of gift authorship in both papers – and, again, a personal tragedy, this time for an eminent and much-liked jovial professor of obstetrics. From the journalological aspect, the editorial processes at the journal were slapdash. The case report had not been peer reviewed by an external assessor, whilst in the second paper the credulity of the referee and of the editors in accepting Pearce's claims in a condition of such rarity (which he repeated when they checked with him) was extraordinary.

Subsequently two further cases of consultants from teaching hospitals, who were also struck off the Medical Register by the GMC, confirmed that Pearce's story was by no means unique: **John Anderton**, an Edinburgh physician and some time registrar of the Royal College of Physicians of Edinburgh, had faked some results in a drug trial (see Chapter 5),[27] as had **Robert Davies**, professor of respiratory medicine at St Bartholomew's Hospital, London.[28] All this led to three editors voicing their concerns (for example, an editorial in the *Lancet*[29]) and the formation of COPE, discussed by my fellow-editor, Michael Farthing, later in this book. Yet another committee was set up at the time of the Edinburgh conference, and at the time of writing it still has to report. (Ironically, also, as I was completing this chapter, the *BMJ* and the *Lancet* had a further editorial from these editors, commenting yet again on the failure of the British medical Establishment to do anything in the 13 months that had elapsed since the Edinburgh meeting).[30] However, to anybody aware of how the Establishment fails to do what it doesn't want to – seen also, for instance, with the failure of the GMC to protect the public by efficient self-regulation of professional standards – the omens for a really worthwhile outcome (an efficient system, with teeth) are not, I think, very positive. I have instanced the way in which this country failed to ensure that proper ethical standards were applied in research involving patients and volunteers. Indeed, for any ancien régime (including France and Germany, where I suspect that the future is also going to be *dolce far niente*) confronted with a paradigm shift, the response is to smile gently and go on in the smug old ways. Not for nothing was it a physician, Wilfred Trotter, who stated that: "The most powerful antigen known to man is a new idea."

References

1 Nimmo WS, ed. Joint consensus conference on misconduct in biomedical research. *Proc R Coll Physicians Edinb* 2000;**30**(Suppl. 7).
2 Kevles DJ. *The Baltimore case: a trial of politics, science, and character.* New York: Norton, 1987.
3 Medawar P. *Advice to a young scientist.* Cambridge: Harper and Row, 1979.
4 Broad W, Wade N. *Betrayers of the truth.* New York: Simon and Schuster, 1982.
5 Kohn A. *False prophets.* Oxford: Blackwell, 1986.
6 Association of American Medical Colleges. *The maintenance of high ethical standards in the conduct of research.* Washington DC: AAMC, 1982.
7 Institute of Medicine. *The responsible conduct of research.* Washington DC: IOM, 1989.
8 Association of American Universities. *Framework for institutional policies and procedures to deal with fraud in research.* Washington DC: AAU, 1988.
9 Majerus P. Fraud in medical research. *J Clin Invest* 1982;**70**:213–17.
10 Relman AS. Lessons from the Darsee affair. *N Engl J Med* 1983;**308**:1415–17.
11 Maddox J. Whose misconduct? *Nature* 1987;**326**:831–2.
12 General Medical Council. Letter from the President, 1 December 1999.
13 LaFollette MC. *Stealing into print.* Berkeley: University of California Press, 1992.
14 Anonymous. Erasures from register. *BMJ* 1975;**2**:392.
15 Miller DJ, Herson M, eds. *Research fraud in the behavioral and biomedical sciences.* New York: Wiley, 1992.
16 Stewart WW, Feder N. The integrity of the scientific literature. *Nature* 1987;**207**:14.
17 Culliton BJ. Harvard researchers retract data in immunology paper. *Science* 1987;**237**:718–19.
18 Kochan CA, Budd JM. The persistence of fraud in the literature: the Darsee case. *J Am Soc Information Sci* 1992;**43**:488–93.
19 Friedman PJ. Research ethics, due process, and common sense. *JAMA* 1988;**260**:1937–8.
20 Sabbagh K. *A Rum affair.* London: Viking, 1999.
21 Swan N. Baron Munchausen at the bedside. In: Lock S, Wells F, eds. *Fraud and misconduct in medical research.* London: BMJ, 1996.
22 Lagarde D, Maisonneuve H. Fraud in clinical research from sample preparation to publication: the French scene. In: Lock S, Wells F, eds. *Fraud and misconduct in medical research.* London: BMJ, 1993.
23 Stegemann-Boehl S. Some legal aspects of misconduct in science: a German view. In: Lock S, Wells F, eds. *Fraud and misconduct in medical research.* London: BMJ, 1996.

24 Royal College of Physicians of London. *Fraud and misconduct in medical research*. London: RCP, 1991.
25 Harvard Medical School. *Faculty policies on integrity in science*. Cambridge, Mass: Faculty of Medicine, Harvard University, 1994.
26 Doyal L, Tobias JS, eds. *Informed consent in medical research*. London: BMJ, 2000.
27 Mitchell P. Edinburgh doctor struck off because of clinical-trial fraud. *Lancet* 1997; 350:272.
28 Dyer C. London professor struck off for bullying and dishonesty. *BMJ* 1999;319:938.
29 Anonymous. Dealing with deception. *Lancet* 1996;347:843.
30 Farthing M, Horton R, Smith R. Research misconduct: Britain's failure to act. *BMJ* 2000;321:1485–6.

5: Counteracting research misconduct: a decade of British pharmaceutical industry action

FRANK WELLS

This book deals in depth with the subject of fraud and misconduct in the context of biomedical research as a whole. This specific chapter deals with the role and experience of the pharmaceutical industry in the UK, now over a period of over 10 years, in preventing, detecting, investigating, and prosecuting such fraud and misconduct. It stands as a stark contrast to the inactivity seen outside the industry and outside the UK.

The welfare of patients is fundamental to the practice of medicine. That there are so many effective treatments available for the cure or control of so many diseases is largely the outcome of decades of research, stretching throughout the second half of the 20th century. Much research must continue, both to improve upon existing treatments and to master diseases including the cancers, psychoses, dementia, and many others, which are currently untreatable successfully. Clinical research therefore remains essential, including genetic and biotechnological research, with the recognition that the interests of patient-subjects involved in such research must be safeguarded. The Declaration of Helsinki sets out the principles of such safeguards, and its regular revision by the World Medical Association emphasises its paramount importance.[1]

Fraud in clinical research can be defined as "the generation of false data with the intent to deceive". This definition includes all of the components of fraud: the making-up of information that does not exist, and intending to do so flagrantly in order to deceive others into believing that the information is true. Exploitation in the context of clinical research is one of the greatest potential hazards to the welfare of individual patients and, indeed, to society as a whole. Such exploitation is rare, though quantifying its actual likelihood remains difficult. There is enough published evidence to confirm that fraud in clinical research is ever-present.[2]

Fraud in any context is deplorable, but if it is primarily prescription, tax, or financial fraud then the only party at risk is the one who loses money – and this may be the Government or, ultimately, the taxpayer. *Research* fraud distorts the database on which many decisions may be made, possibly adversely affecting thousands of others. *Clinical* research fraud is potentially even more dangerous: if licensing decisions regarding medicines were to be made based on efficacy and safety data that are false, the result could be disastrous. Furthermore, individual patients may be the unwitting victims, believing that the unexpectedly frequent and intensive care that they are receiving – including numerous blood tests, ECGs and other investigations – demonstrate dedication on the part of the doctor, whereas they are being flagrantly exploited without them realising it. The importance of the roles of both the clinical trial monitor and the independent auditor in this regard cannot be overemphasised. Nevertheless they are inadequate by themselves: when a fraudster is determined to cheat and to cover his tracks, auditors are hoodwinked into believing that all is well.

Ideally, fraud should not occur – but we do not live in an ideal world; agreed high standards must be set for clinical research, to which all interested parties should adhere. However, procedures must also be in place if misconduct is suspected despite the existence of these standards. Within the pharmaceutical industry, the standards needed for the conduct of clinical research already exist, and have been adopted by all the regulatory bodies who license medicines, international pharmaceutical companies and contract research organisations. Both the European Commission (CPMP) Good Clinical Practice (GCP) guidelines[3] and the requirements of the FDA came first, but GCP guidelines, adopted under the International Conference on Harmonisation (ICH) process,[4] now take precedence, globally. The Step 5 stage having been reached, there is now global guidance – which means that there are now global standards – that have been adopted by the three major sectors of Europe, the USA, and Japan. A European Commission directive on clinical research will soon be operative throughout Europe, once individual member states have adopted it, thus giving the force of law to the ICH GCP agreement. Although the standards referred to above are therefore in place, there is no such harmonisation when it comes to dealing with fraud and misconduct in the context of clinical research. Indeed, even within Europe there is as yet no agreed attitude towards tackling the problem.

Fraud is much less common than carelessness, although, as indicated above, its incidence is difficult to quantify. Lock has referred to the various estimates that been made[5] but, based on the work on cases of fraud in which I have been involved during the last 10 years, my personal belief is that it is at least 1%. If we accept this figure of 1%, this means that, in the UK where I am based, maybe 30 studies are being conducted at any one time that could be fraudulent. Extrapolating this to the rest of the world – and there is no evidence that the incidence of fraud in clinical research differs across Europe or North America (although we are more open in dealing with it in the UK) – then there may be between 125 and 150 clinical trials being

65

conducted, now, where some of the data being generated are fraudulent, where investigators are making up some of the data to be submitted to a company and – worst of all – may be exploiting their patients in the process. But, whatever its incidence, this unacceptable aspect of clinical research must be tackled if we are to achieve and maintain confidence in scientific integrity and in the clinical research process.

Historical aspect of fraud

This aspect is dealt with comprehensively in the resumé chapter by Lock, but reference must be made to the role of the trade association for the pharmaceutical industry in the UK, the Association of the British Pharmaceutical Industry (ABPI) in advising on the management of potential fraud in research during the past decade. One particular aspect of the problem, which has puzzled outside observers is that there is so little mention of clinical research fraud in the literature coming from the pharmaceutical industry. However, until the early 1990s in the UK and still persisting even now elsewhere, pharmaceutical companies suspecting fraud were greatly concerned about the risk of recrimination, adverse publicity, and loss of favour, support and, indeed, prescriptions, if they were seen to be critical of the medical profession. These concerns had some justification: in one particular case, where, following fraud, the name of the doctor was struck from the Medical Register, the company that had been defrauded was boycotted by the doctors in the district, albeit only temporarily.[6] Nevertheless, these concerns have been overcome in the UK and it was in 1992 that the ABPI set up a working party on misconduct in clinical research, following the publication of a report by the Royal College of Physicians on fraud and misconduct in medical research,[7] on which it seemed that little action would follow. This was against a background of increasing confidence on the part of pharmaceutical companies to take action against doctors found to have submitted fraudulent data, but who were uncertain how best to investigate or to handle suspicions that such data might be fraudulent.

The working party recognised that what was needed was a mechanism that could make it easier for member companies to pursue such suspicions without prejudice. Details of the procedures to be adopted by companies are set out in Chapter 6 by Brock.

One of the most frequently reported problems arising from the detection of suspected fraud was deciding what to do with the information that has been gathered – and outside the UK and the four Nordic countries this situation still exists. Might there be other cases of suspected fraud that other companies had detected from the same investigator? It would hardly be right and proper to contact other companies at random to raise such queries, and, at the very least, company pharmaceutical physicians might fear that they were laying themselves open to the laws of libel or defamation if they suggested to others that a doctor might be acting fraudulently.

The ABPI working party considered this at length because no mechanism then existed in the UK or, for that matter, elsewhere, to enable such doubts to be shared outside the company in which the doubts had been generated. It concluded that it was in the public interest for pharmaceutical physicians to report to an independent third party any serious concerns that they might have, in good faith, regarding a specific investigator.[8] The way forward, on which legal advice was taken, was to invest in the ABPI, and specifically in the ABPI medical director, a "possibly suspect doctor name-holding" responsibility. The medical director of a company can ask the ABPI medical director whether the name of a possibly suspect doctor had already been reported by another company, and be given the answer "yes" or "no". No list is promulgated (other than of those doctors who have already gone through the full disciplinary machinery of the General Medical Council (GMC) and been found guilty of serious professional misconduct, who have been prosecuted in the courts and found guilty, or whose names are on the list promulgated by the Food and Drug Administration of the USA). On a doctor-to-doctor basis, the name of the company medical director who first provided the ABPI with evidence of suspicion about an investigator is given to the company medical director making a subsequent inquiry with similar evidence of suspicion. The ABPI medical director is also in a position to advise companies when, in his opinion, evidence reported from more than one company has, when accumulated, created a strong enough case to submit to the GMC, even if the evidence from one company alone did not. A round table discussion may then be held, particularly when more than two companies are suspicious of the same investigator, as has happened now on a number of occasions.

This arrangement, within the industry, works well in the UK – as the following case histories clearly demonstrate – but a similar arrangement needs to operate outside the industry, and outside the UK. Chapters 8, 9 and 10 from the Nordic countries set out the highly successful schemes in those countries, whereby an independent body (or, now, bodies in Denmark), inspiring the confidence of the whole scientific fraternity, can investigate any case of suspected scientific dishonesty; this could be taken as a model on which similar arrangements could be adopted in other countries, including the UK. A consensus conference held in Edinburgh in 1999 under the auspices of the Royal College of Physicians of Edinburgh and of the Faculty of Pharmaceutical Medicine addressed this issue and concluded that what should happen next should be the establishment of a national panel – with public representation – to provide advice and assistance on request[9] but, as has happened time and again, the outcome of this conclusion has yet to materialise. Whereas the doctor sequentially occupying the post of ABPI medical director *has* fulfilled the role described with moderate success, it would be preferable to have in place an independent body to take on an advisory role for cases outside, as well as inside, industry-sponsored clinical trials; in practical terms any subsequent investigatory role can, currently uniquely, if funded, be conducted by an independent commercial agency. The activities of the only one currently conducting such investigations are described in Chapter 16 by Jay.

The prosecution of fraud

Once an investigator has been shown beyond all reasonable shadow of doubt to have submitted fraudulent data to a pharmaceutical company or contract house, it is essential in the interests of the public, the profession, and the industry that that doctor should be dealt with. In the UK this is usually by referral to the General Medical Council (GMC) for possible consideration by the professional conduct committee. Alternatively, the doctor may be prosecuted for the criminal offence of deception. Chapter 16 by Jay deals with the GMC procedure and other legal issues.

The following cases are typical examples of those submitted by pharmaceutical companies in conjunction with the ABPI to the General Medical Council.

The case of the Durham psychiatrist

During 1986, Reckitt and Colman undertook a clinical trial on a new antidepressant medicine, for which it required a number of consultant psychiatrist investigators. One such doctor, much respected in Durham, the city where he was employed as a hospital consultant, was Dr VA Siddiqui.[6]

This doctor presented all the data needed for the 15 patients he had entered into a clinical trial following a long session one Saturday afternoon when he had sat down and invented much of it. The record forms were all too neat, and were all submitted at the same time; this raised doubts in the mind of the CRA, and thence of the medical adviser, in charge of the trial. This doctor happened to be one of a number of consultants taking part in a pivotal study for a new tricyclic antidepressant – sadly, unbeknown to the CRA, he was involved in seven other trials at the same time, many of them potentially sharing the same patient population. The local ethics research committee had expressed mild surprise that he had submitted so many trial protocols for approval, but had never queried whether he could manage them all at the same time. His reputation in his home city was one of great dedication to duty.

When the data arrived, unexpectedly complete in view of the recruitment difficulties that the doctor had reported, the CRA went to great lengths to check the source data, and found considerable difficulty in doing so. For some reason, the doctor chose to refer his haematology and biochemistry specimens to two different laboratories – one in Durham and one in Bishop Auckland. Neither laboratory had any data at all for one patient, but both laboratories had some data for all the other patients, but not what the investigator had submitted to the company. When challenged by the medical adviser, he denied that he had fabricated any of the information, claiming that, under stress at the time, he had handed the management of this particular trial to his registrar. He could not remember her name, and she had now left. At this stage the Regional Health Authority was asked for its help – not to investigate a possible crime, because there was no evidence of harm to any patients – but to supply the name and new address of the registrar. She was written to by the company at this address, several hundred miles away, and in her reply she indignantly and forthrightly denied that she had had anything whatsoever to do with her previous consultant's research projects. Because he had so many, she and her colleagues never had time to do anything other than look after all the NHS patients who, she implied, rather suffered from her erstwhile chief's involvement in other things.

The case was a strong one, and the ABPI assisted the member pharmaceutical company to bring the doctor's activities to the attention of the General Medical Council by means of a simple statutory declaration. The case was considered by the professional conduct committee. The doctor concerned was found guilty of serious professional misconduct, and his name was erased from the Medical Register.

The immediate aftermath was most unfortunate. Because there was no local mechanism for investigating this sort of misconduct, no one locally knew anything about it, and the doctor involved certainly did not talk about it. When the news broke that evening, the local paper carried banner headlines – and the local medical community was horrified and incredulous. How dare the ABPI and a pharmaceutical company do this to one of their highly respected colleagues? That was the last time they would have anything to do with that particular company, and they banned the company from access to the Postgraduate Medical Centre forthwith. Fortunately, the Regional Medical Officer and the Clinical Tutor agreed to a meeting with the ABPI, which was held on site in Durham, at which it was possible to relate the facts – specifically the iniquities of the doctor and the integrity of the GMC – to representatives of the local doctors. The status quo ante was restored as a result, but the immediate effect had been disastrous.

There is no doubt that this was a pivotal case. Despite the initial adverse response, on reflection it was appreciated that appropriate action had indeed been taken against a doctor who had fabricated data, falsified the results of a clinical trial, and exploited both his patients and the pharmaceutical company. It was realised that any pharmaceutical company that did *not* take action against a doctor committing fraud or research misconduct would itself be vulnerable; the media had praised the company for its action, once the facts were fully revealed, and could be expected to pillory a company that did not pursue a similar policy in similar circumstances.

The case of the Plaistow practitioner

In Autumn 1990 Fisons contracted with Data Analysis and Research (DAR) Limited, of Cambridge, to undertake a multicentre clinical trial entitled "An open crossover study to compare the acceptability and efficacy of Tilade Mint (4 mg qds) delivered by the Autohaler with Tilade Mint (4 mg qds) delivered by the standard metered dose inhaler".

Fisons suggested to DAR that, amongst others, Dr RB Gonsai, a single-handed general practitioner in Plaistow, London, E13, might have an interest in this trial. DAR wrote to him enquiring as to whether he would be interested in participating in the trial, enclosing a form on which he was to indicate his interest or disinterest, and a summary of the protocol. He completed and returned this form confirming his interest. He was visited two months later by a DAR clinical research associate to discuss the trial, following which he was confirmed as a suitable potential investigator.

An initiation meeting was held six months later, at which the study design was again discussed with a detailed review of the case record forms. At that meeting Dr Gonsai signed a formal agreement to participate in the trial, the protocol, an indemnity letter, and a receipt for the investigator brochure. These documents clearly stated that the trial was to be monitored by authorised individuals with respect to current guidelines on Good Clinical (Research) Practice. Clinical supplies and documentation were provided for five patients.

A routine monitoring telephone call to Dr Gonsai was made after one month, at which he confirmed he had recruited four patients, although he had not returned their enrolment cards. During this telephone call, an appointment was made for a monitoring visit the following week, but 24 hours before the appointment, when a call was made to confirm it, Dr Gonsai cancelled the appointment, and it did not prove possible to hold the first monitoring meeting until one full month later. At that meeting the data for the four patients were reviewed. For one patient, the documentation appeared satisfactory. The data for the other three patients revealed an anomaly regarding the dates of assessments: the third assessments for each of these three patients were all dated *in advance of* the monitoring visit.

Dr Gonsai explained that his wife, who helped with completion of the clinical report forms, had dated these assessment forms in advance, but that the appointments book confirmed that the patients had visited the surgery earlier, although verification with the NHS notes of these patients revealed no record of these visits having taken place.

Regarding the diary cards, required to be completed by each patient, further anomalies arose. The entries for two of the four patients were *completed* for up to two weeks in advance of the monitoring visit. Dr Gonsai could offer no explanation for this.

A further monitoring appointment was made so that the company might seek a written explanation from Dr Gonsai on the completion of diary cards by patients beyond the dates of their last visits, and to check the appointments book. This appointment was duly fulfilled early in September 1991, when it was noted that Dr Gonsai had recruited one further patient into the study.

A number of further issues were raised, which required clarification at a subsequent meeting.

1   For the fifth recruited patient no diary cards were available at all. Dr Gonsai stated that the patient had not returned them, and additionally that he had issued old cards to the patient, from a previous study.
2   The FEV and FVC values were identical for all three visits for three patients, and for two visits for the fourth and fifth patients. These results are beyond reasonable bounds of statistical coincidence.
3   The evening peak flow readings recorded by one patient were outside the range of the peak flow meter.
4   The morning and evening peak flow readings were identical for all patients on all the diary cards; there is usually a variation between morning and evening readings in real life, and the chances of finding this constant uniformity of data in practice are beyond belief.
5   The contract house queried further the state of the diary cards. They were in pristine condition, without any of the usual evidence of handling found on their return from patient use. It was also queried why two sets of the diary cards appeared to be in the same handwriting, and, again, why some of the data had been completed on diary cards beyond the date of the final visit of the patient to the doctor.

On the strong grounds of probability, it was concluded that the data submitted by Dr Gonsai to DAR included entries that were incompatible with the facts concerning the patients to whom they were supposed to refer, and that this constituted serious professional misconduct, justifying referral to the General Medical Council. At a hearing before the Professional Conduct Committee Dr Gonsai was indeed found guilty of serious professional misconduct, and his name was erased from the Medical Register.

The case of the GP from Glasgow

In February 1991 the Astra Clinical Research Unit set up a four-centre general practitioner clinical trial in Glasgow, designed to compare felodipine ER once daily with nifedipine SR twice daily given as monotherapy for the treatment of patients with mild to moderate hypertension. One of these four centres was Dr David Latta's practice. The data submitted to the company by Dr Latta during the course of this trial were so at variance with what would be expected, and with what were in fact submitted by the other centres, that a source verification audit was conducted.

The following results were obtained:

1   All 22 patients had exactly 100% compliance.
2   All 22 patients had returned all the empty blister packs in which the trial medication was supplied.
3   All 22 patients had kept drug boxes in pristine condition.
4   21 of the 22 patients had period lengths on treatment of exactly 28 days.

5   All 22 patients completed quality-of-life questionnaires, and all were in pristine condition. There were no changes of mind or mistakes in the questionnaires.

6   No patients in the study reported any adverse experiences.

7   No patients withdrew from the study, and all 22 patients completed the study as per protocol.

8   The range of BP readings was extremely small, and an exceptionally large proportion of patients maintained a heart rate of 74.
    (All the above points were not in accord with usual trial experience, in which considerable variation in patient behaviour is seen, and this in itself raised suspicion. However, subsequent points were of greater concern.)

9   Most of the blood test results were on forms which had had the patient's name or sample date cut off the source document. Some of the documents had been stamped by the laboratory with a date preceding the date on which the sample was supposed to have been taken; some of these dates had been altered in pen to the correct date.

10 The doctor claimed to have used pseudonyms for the samples he submitted, but had forgotten them, and so copies of the damaged laboratory report forms could not be obtained.

11 Some of the damaged laboratory report forms appeared to have been signed by a doctor who had left the laboratory in December 1990, three months before the first patient was recruited.

12 The consent forms were all produced retrospectively and a number of these forms appeared to have been signed by the same hand.

13 No record of any of the patient data generated during the course of the trial was entered into the patients' NHS records; separate NHS record cards were generated, retrospectively, from data recorded in the clinical trial record forms, some in the presence of the trial monitor. These were therefore meaningless as source data.

14 The ECGs for eight patients appeared identical; for a further four patients they appeared differently identical; and for a further seven patients again appeared identical. This implies that for 19 patients just three ECG tracings were used.

15 The study file had not been used, and no record of drug accountability was taken.

The sum total of the above was so at variance with what would be expected that it was highly likely on the grounds of probability that some of the data generated by Dr Latta in this trial was fraudulent, and the evidence was therefore submitted to the General Medical Council. At a hearing before the Professional Conduct Committee, Dr Latta was found guilty of serious professional misconduct, and his name was erased from the Medical Register.

The case of the partners in Leeds

During 1989, a contract research organisation was commissioned by three different pharmaceutical companies to undertake a series of clinical trials in general practice. The first of these was on a new product for the treatment of hypertension; the second was a multicentre paediatric asthma trial; and the third was also a multicentre trial on a product for the treatment of asthma.[10]

The contract research company recruited Drs CJ Chandnani and CJ Vishin, in partnership in Rothwell, Leeds, amongst others, to take part in these trials, both these doctors having previously conducted clinical trials for the organisation, and with which no unsatisfactory features had been associated. The doctors signed formal agreements with the organisation on accepting, on each occasion, the conditions applying to the conduct of the three different trials.

The first trial required, amongst other things, the completion of diary cards by the patients. However, the completion of these cards gave rise to suspicion, and as a result Dr Chandnani was visited by the quality assurance manager. The handwriting on the diary cards was remarkably similar to that of Dr Chandnani, and they were in pristine condition, unlike those of the patients of the other investigators in the trial, which showed the expected signs of frequent handling.

When asked how he had obtained such good records, in similar handwriting to his own, Dr Chandnani stated that he was very careful to instruct patients on the correct method of completing diary cards, that none of his patients had requested his advice in completing the cards, and that they had not copied his handwriting.

One patient had apparently completed the diary card for an extra seven days, during which time the card was actually in the possession of the company. Dr Chandnani's explanation that his patient must have turned over two pages at once and then crossed them out and entered them on the correct page was not substantiated by close examination of the diary card. The circumstantial evidence pointed to the diary cards having been completed by Dr Chandnani himself.

In the second trial, diary cards completed by patients were also used. Patients had to record the daily medication, and the times when it was taken, severity of asthma symptoms and daily morning and evening peak flow readings measured by three successive "blows" each time. According to the age of the patients involved, the recording on diary cards was either by the patient, a parent, guardian or friend.

The data for all the patients recruited by Drs Chandnani and Vishin were completed with the minimum of delay, which indicated rapid recruitment and rapid completion of the study.

Later in 1990, the contract research organisation was contacted about another study by a different company and Dr Chandnani again agreed to participate. As with the paediatric asthma study, he recruited all his patients very quickly. One patient, however, was noted to be a protocol violator, as the monitor found that the initials of this one patient were the same as a patient participating in a safety study for a third pharmaceutical company, and it turned out that these two patients were indeed one and the same.

The pattern of data recorded by Drs Chandnani and Vishin in this trial differed considerably from the pattern observed by the other investigators taking part in the same study; the variability in the readings of morning peak flow measurements from the patients of Drs Chandnani and Vishin were markedly less than the considerable variability in readings from all the other patients. With regard to Dr Chandnani's patients, they were all purported to have recorded peak flow readings to the nearest "2", which is not within the sensitivity of the instrument recording peak flow, and such accuracy was not the case for any other patients – including those of Dr Vishin – who recorded to the nearest "5" or "10".

With regard to the handwriting on some of the patient diary cards, these again showed a marked similarity to the handwriting of Dr Chandnani himself. He characteristically used a "double dot" after writing initials, and there were many examples of the "double dot" phenomenon in the diary cards purported to have been completed by his patients.

In the third study, the contract house trial director was alarmed by the conduct of Drs Chandnani and Vishin in the other two studies, and made a particular point of monitoring all aspects of the study very closely. He found that patient recruitment and attendance for review had been much better than would be expected, and than had been demonstrated at other centres involved in this particular trial. He also examined the trial materials returned by the two doctors and found that unused tablets had been returned in containers showing no signs of wear and tear. Consequently, data were extracted from the case record forms for statistical examination. Scatter plots were produced and compared with data from other investigators in the study. The data from the suspect investigators demonstrated blood pressure readings much more consistent than would be expected with normal variation, in distinct contrast to the data from other investigators.

Most serious and conclusive of all, blood samples, which had been taken for other purposes, were assayed for the investigational drug and its metabolites and these could not identified in samples provided by Drs Chandnani and Vishin. Samples from other investigators were also analysed and showed good correlation with the expected intake of the trial drug. So it was proved beyond all shadow of doubt that the patients had not taken the product at times they were supposed to have taken it, if at all.

Much of the above evidence was circumstantial at the time, but documents were subsequently found, which substantiated all the points made. Further investigation confirmed that some of the patients of Drs Chandnani and Vishin were not involved in the studies mentioned above in which they were purported to have taken part. The sum total of the evidence led to the inevitable conclusion that both these doctors had acted fraudulently, which justified their referral to the General Medical Council.

At a hearing before the Professional Conduct Committee, Drs Chandnani and Vishin were found guilty of serious professional misconduct, and their names were erased from the Medical Register.

The case of the Liverpool GP

In 1990 and early 1991 a pharmaceutical company undertook a multicentre Phase II/III clinical trial, intended as a pivotal registration study, for the treatment of perennial allergic rhinoconjunctivitis. The trial was conducted to standards of Good Clinical Research Practice, and included an assessment of haematology and biochemistry; patients were required to complete diary cards.[10]

The company recruited a number of general practitioners to conduct this study including a Dr P Daengsvang of Liverpool. Dr Daengsvang had previously participated in another study carried out by the company, and his conduct of this previous study had been satisfactory. He was approached again by the company and asked if he would be interested in taking part in this new study, and, having studied the protocol, he signed an agreement to follow the procedures outlined in the protocol. He also signed a financial agreement and was visited by the clinical trial monitor and given supplies of documents and trial medication for him to recruit 15 patients.

Dr Daengsvang recruited patients so quickly that he requested, and was granted, facilities to recruit an additional 10 patients. Within 10 weeks he had recruited a total of 20 patients, and was eventually visited again by the clinical trial monitor to collect the completed case record forms and residual trial material. The company review of the returned record forms raised suspicion because of the uncommon cleanliness of the patient diaries and the "perfection" of the study data. A comparison was made with the progress and results in the other centres taking part in the study.

From a site audit conducted at Dr Daengsvang's surgery and the comparative review, conclusions were reached as noted in Table 5.1.

Table 5.1 Conclusions from site audit and comparative review.

1. Number of patients enrolled, and eligibility

	No. enrolled	No. eligible after run-in
Other centres	148	112
Dr Daengsvang	20	20

It is highly unlikely that this difference is due to chance ($P = 0.008$)

2. Patients completing one month's treatment

	No. eligible	No. completed
Other centres	112	83
Dr Daengsvang	20	20

It is highly unlikely that this difference is due to chance ($P = 0.007$)

3. Change in haemoglobin from entry to the end of the study

	Change of $< 2g/dl$	Change of $> 2g/dl$
Other centres	83	1
Dr Daengsvang	14	6

It is highly unlikely that this difference is due to chance ($P < 0.001$)

The company next submitted photocopies of the consent forms allegedly signed by the 20 patients recruited by Dr Daengsvang, and 19 original patient diaries to the Division of Questioned Documents of the Laboratory of the Government Chemist.

The conclusions were:

- The patient entries on a number of diaries were probably written by one person.
- The entries were unlikely to have been written on a daily basis.
- The authentic writing of Dr Daengsvang shows similarities with the patient entries in 16 of the diaries.

The audit at Dr Daengsvang's surgery yielded the following relevant details:

- The NHS records of at least four patients indicated that they had been seen by the doctor on the alleged study dates but for reasons not related to the study.
- For one study patient the NHS record date of birth had been altered from 1914 to 1974. However, the recorded medical history and living circumstances corresponded to a patient aged 76, not a patient aged 16.

The case was considered at length, and it was concluded that Dr Daengsvang violated the protocol for this trial:

- by using real patients as phantom subjects in the trial, possibly requiring some of them to have unnecessary blood tests;
- by using post-treatment blood samples taken from different subjects than at entry to the study;
- by tampering with NHS records so as to provide spurious source document verification;
- by completing some of the patient diaries himself; and
- by generating false data on certain case report forms,

and in so doing demonstrated serious professional misconduct, justifying referral to the General Medical Council.

At a hearing before the Professional Conduct Committee, heard in his absence, Dr Daengsvang was found guilty of serious professional misconduct, and his name was erased from the Medical Register.

The case of the challenged company

In 1996 a pharmaceutical physician moved from the French subsidiary of an international company to a different company in England. On his arrival in the UK he shared with the managing director of the company he had just joined his concerns that the data accompanying a marketing authorisation submission to a national licensing authority were incomplete, leaving out some of the adverse reactions that had been reported during certain clinical trials, the positive (efficacy) results of which had been included in their entirety. Clearly the doctor felt strongly that he should whistleblow in this case, with which his new managing director concurred. However, the managing director recommended that the facts should be fully ascertained first and the case was therefore next referred to MedicoLegal Investigations.

These began by interviewing the research director of the parent company of the French subsidiary so as to secure his complete cooperation and his confidence in what MLI would be investigating. The medical director and chief executive of the subsidiary company were then interviewed and the safety information within the dossier submitted to the licensing authority was reviewed. It became apparent that the dossier clearly included the complete safety data arising from all the clinical trials referenced in the dossier, as well as the efficacy data. The grounds for the whistleblower's concerns were thus not confirmed. Further enquiries confirmed that no other studies had been conducted on the investigational substance in question, and there was therefore no suggestion that the overall picture regarding the product might have been distorted by any selection of studies to be included in the submission. However, it also became clear that, for reasons which never became entirely clear, though likely to be related to why the doctor chose to change companies at this stage in his career, the whistleblower had not had access to the final dossier submitted to the licensing authority.

It was accepted that the whistleblower had acted in good faith, even though his concerns were unfounded. The company concerned accepted that, for itself, it had learned from this episode that it needed to ensure that those who had responsibility for compiling the safety and efficacy data for a marketing authorisation submission were fully informed regarding the contents of the final submission. The pharmaceutical physician involved has since moved on from his post in the UK.

The case of the Norwood GP

In March 1993 a company commenced a randomised double blind placebo controlled multicentre clinical trial in both hospital and general practice on the efficacy of a new treatment for severe depression. Soon after, another company commenced the UK component of a randomised double blind multinational clinical trial on the effects of a new medicine on high risk patients with hypertension.[11]

One of the investigators chosen for both studies, though quite independently, was Dr James Bochsler, a single handed general practitioner in Upper Norwood, South London. He had not previously conducted any research for the first company, but had expressed an interest in taking part to one of the company field force representatives, to whom he had also stated that he had done a number of studies previously for other companies. He had, indeed, previously conducted research for the second company and had been selected to take part in the hypertension study according to that company's strict criteria.

With regard to the first study, on a treatment for depression, setting-up the study centre for Dr Bochsler took some time, as he had to be issued with the guidance to investigators booklet published by the ABPI, to attend a preliminary investigators' meeting and to satisfy the company that he was prepared to conduct the clinical trial in accordance with these guidelines. This was done, and he duly signed an agreement, which included a commitment to conduct the study strictly in accordance with the principles contained within the Declaration of Helsinki. At the investigators' meeting he had expressed unhappiness at the prospect of direct source document (medical record) verification (SDV) by the company monitor and he was reluctant to obtain Local Research Ethics Committee approval, but both these concerns were overcome.

Dr Bochsler duly started the trial and monitoring visits began. To begin with, it appeared from these monitoring visits that recruitment was very good, and that data recording, drug accountability, and source document verification were satisfactory. However, suspicions soon began to be raised. First, a large number of patient assessments, which were clearly missing on the first day of a monitoring visit, had all mysteriously appeared by the following day. Next, medication bottles, which should have been issued to all of these patients, if they had attended for assessments on the due dates, were still present in Dr Bochsler's surgery. When challenged, he alleged that the patients, whose medication was still in the surgery, had been withdrawn from the study for administrative reasons. The opportunity was taken to obtain photocopies of all the signed consent forms, as Dr Bochsler appeared to have seen a number of patients when, according to the practice appointments book and diary, he was on holiday.

The situation was investigated further and a number of patients were interviewed. Several patients confirmed that they had not given consent to take part in a study, and at least one patient did not appear to exist.

With regard to the second study, on a treatment for hypertension, routine monitoring took place and, again, it appeared at first that recruitment was good, and that data recording, drug accountability, and source document verification were satisfactory. Dr Bochsler was selected routinely for audit, as part of standard company practice. Suspicions then became roused. In particular, these included electrocardiogram tracings (ECGs), which had been duplicated and re-assigned to different patients; and returned medication, which appeared in pristine condition apart from crushing of the outer packaging of each box in a similar fashion. Similarities in handwriting for the signatures of certain patients was noted on the consent forms, which were duly photocopied. Further investigations were therefore conducted, and a number of patients were interviewed, many of them confirming that the signatures on the consent forms purporting to be theirs were clearly forgeries.

Both cases were submitted to the General Medical Council as examples of serious professional misconduct, and at a hearing of the professional conduct committee Dr Bochsler's name was erased from the Medical Register. Standard GMC procedure is to allow 28 days to elapse during which time the doctor may consider an appeal before erasure takes place but, unusually, this erasure was with immediate effect, as the professional conduct committee felt that the offences were so serious that the chance of their being repeated had to be stopped at once.

The cases of two doctors who died

In September 1994 a major international pharmaceutical company commenced a randomised multinational multicentre comparative Phase IV clinical trial on the effects of a new formulation of an established medicine on high risk patients with hypertension. The company arranged that the UK component of this trial should be supervised by a contract research organisation. The study divided patients into two treatment groups in a randomised double blind fashion involving treatment for a total of three years.[12]

One of the investigators chosen was a GP whose surgery was located in a rural village. He had previously conducted research for the contract research organisation and other companies, and was considered an experienced investigator. He signed the protocol, the investigators' agreement and the financial agreement. Monitoring visits were subsequently conducted by clinical research associates from the contract research organisation, but they experienced considerable difficulty in arranging the necessary visits with the doctor. When eventually a visit took place certain discrepancies were noted. These included the presence of trial medication for several patients, which was purported to have been dispensed, entries included in the clinical report forms for dates when the doctor was allegedly on holiday, and the absence of any correlation between the NHS notes for three patients and their purported clinical trial record forms.

A further monitoring visit three weeks later confirmed that medication reported in the record forms for certain patients as having been supplied had not been dispensed, as the drugs were still present, unopened, at the surgery premises. The irregularities noted on these two monitoring visits were reported to the sponsoring company. After some difficulty in arranging a confirmed date, in part attributable to the doctor's purported vacation in Italy, when he was in fact at home, an audit visit was made. A subsequent audit visit was made one month later and both audits revealed more discrepancies. Over and above the irregularities noted by the clinical trial monitor, it now appeared that certain original NHS notes had been removed and replaced with study specific information only.

The company concluded that a number of issues had not been satisfactorily explained, and that it was not possible to know to what extent the patients identified by the doctor in this clinical trial had participated. The case was then referred to the ABPI for comment, and thence to MedicoLegal Investigations. Certain further investigations were therefore conducted, and the services of a handwriting analyst were engaged. The evidence from the handwriting analyst, Mr MG Hall, concluded that the signatures of 17 patients on the consent forms and of 17 witnesses, also on the consent forms, were similar to the handwriting of the doctor. Five patients were interviewed, and they confirmed that they had not been asked to take part in this study, that the signatures on the consent forms were not theirs, and therefore forgeries, and some of the witnesses' signatures were also forgeries.

The case was referred to the General Medical Council, but was never heard because the doctor died before any hearing could take place. The circumstances of his death may be relevant to his involvement in not only this study but also a large number of other studies where irregularities were subsequently discovered, including the falsification of trial results and the forging of patient signatures in over 150 patient consent forms. The doctor was aware that this incriminating evidence, which had been hidden away, had been found and that these several further cases were also under forensic investigation. However, all these investigations came to an abrupt halt when the doctor was found dead in the bottom of his swimming pool. The post-mortem report indicated that the doctor had drowned and the coroner returned an open verdict.

The other doctor who died was a partner in a general practice in the Cotswolds. The question of fraud as far as he was concerned first came to light when he admitted to one of his partners that he was suicidal, and that one of the reasons why was that he had fabricated some of the data for a number of clinical trials in which he was involved as an investigator. Professional help was provided for the doctor, but despite this, and being rested from work, some weeks later he committed suicide.

Several features came to light after his death. Firstly, the triggering factor to his admitting to fraud to his partners was probably that he had been found out by at least one of the companies sponsoring a study. This occurred when the chairman of the local research ethics committee discovered that the doctor had sent to this company an approval letter, purporting to come from the committee, which was forged. No submission for this trial had ever been received, let alone considered, by the committee and clearly no letter of approval could possibly have been issued.

The magnitude of his fraudulent activities did not become apparent to anyone until after his death. His former partners needed to ensure that any patients who had been involved in his research activities, whether fraudulent or not, were adequately safeguarded. This proved to be exceedingly difficult, as the doctor had seemingly generated medical records solely for the purposes of source document verification, which he showed to the various clinical trial monitors, but had not indicated anything about clinical trial involvement in the main practice records, which were computerised. Virtually none of the patients, who were ostensibly subjects in these various clinical trials, were aware of their so-called involvement, but neither did most of them receive any study medication. The consent forms were either forged or signed at the doctor's behest for other purposes. Most of the trial supplies were disposed of down the toilet, but the doctor went to sufficient trouble to make it appear that drug reconciliation was reasonable. He arranged for visits from clinical trial monitors always to be held after surgery hours when no patients would be present, nor any other members of the practice partnership or staff. Apparently he kept his partners aware of his interest in research by doing the occasional study authentically, but kept them in the dark about most of his study activities, including those he had fabricated, and consequently kept for himself the payments he subsequently received.

Several observations arise from this case. As an aside, it can be noted that the forging of research ethics committee approval is not unique, as the experience of Blunt referred to elsewhere in this book (Chapter 13) confirms. The pharmaceutical companies concerned were identified only after a considerable amount of detective work, and were dismayed that they themselves had not detected anything suspicious that required further investigation. However, the doctor had clearly gone to considerable lengths to conceal what he was doing, and in my experience fraudsters such as he are classic confidence tricksters, appearing to their patients, their partners and colleagues, and the sponsors of research to be totally beyond reproach. Because all the correspondence between the doctor and the sponsoring companies or contract research organisations had used his home address, and because the trial agreements had been solely between the doctor and the sponsoring company, his partners were quite unaware of the extent of his involvement in clinical trials. If they had been, they might have had a controlling influence, although they might have been surprised that the local research ethics committee was seemingly allowing him to do so much research at the same time – unaware that he was bypassing such approval by forging it.

It should therefore be an accepted policy, enshrined in company standard operating procedures, that agreements involving general practitioner investigators should include a signed statement from or on behalf of any other partners that the practice as a whole is satisfied with the arrangements made for the conduct of that particular study at that particular site. Correspondence should ideally be addressed to the investigator at the practice premises, and monitoring visits should always be made on the actual site where the patient-subjects are being seen. The same principles apply to hospital-based studies, where it should go without saying that an agreement must be signed by the relevant authorities as well as by the investigator.

The case of the Scottish academic nephrologist

In mid-1992, the major international company, Pfizer, decided to conduct a double blind placebo-controlled parallel group clinical trial assessing the safety and efficacy of a new medicine in patients with heart failure and impaired renal function, inadequately controlled on the treatment that they had been taking, unaltered, for at least eight weeks.[13]

One of the investigators chosen by Pfizer to conduct this study was Dr John Anderton, a consultant general physician with a known interest in

81

renal medicine, who was based at the Western General Hospital, Edinburgh. He had previously conducted a number of other studies for the company and was recognised as a distinguished doctor who had previously served as an office-holder of one of the medical royal colleges. The protocol and the usual agreements were signed by both parties; specifically, Dr Anderton agreed to conduct the study as described in the protocol, carried out in conformance with the Declaration of Helsinki, including the obtaining of informed consent from all participating subjects.

Recruitment and assessment of patients for this study appeared satisfactory to start with, but, during a routine visit at which the hospital notes were being checked against entries in the study report forms, the clinical trial monitor suddenly noticed that several patient signatures on the study consent forms were not consistent with patient signatures elsewhere in the hospital notes. The company arranged for two audits to be carried out at Dr Anderton's centre and a number of irregularities were discovered, which are set out below. As a result of these irregularities having been brought to light over this study, Pfizer decided to review the work previously conducted by Dr Anderton on its behalf, and found a number of additional acts of misconduct.

The case was referred to MedicoLegal Investigations and a number of witnesses were interviewed. It was clear that several of the recruited patients were not aware that they had been put into a clinical trial and that their consent had not been sought, let alone obtained. Dr Anderton's personal assistant had also been required, by Dr Anderton, to sign that she had witnessed patients' signatures, which did not, in fact, exist. These are the acts of misconduct committed by Dr Anderton in the course of the two Pfizer studies:

- All the echocardiogram and nuclear medicine data for patients were provided on forms that were no longer used in their respective departments. There was no evidence that the information on these forms had ever been generated by the departments concerned. Dr Anderton, when challenged, admitted that these data were bogus but attributed them to a research fellow working with him at the time, but the research fellow appears to have been invented as Dr Anderton had no records on him, no CV, no forwarding address, and no previous (or subsequent) correspondence.
- Records had been made of the involvement of some patients, and of the effects of their randomly allocated treatment, before they had actually been put on such treatment.
- There were discrepancies between the case report forms and the information given in letters to general practitioners of a number of patients. The letters revealed that the patients' treatment had been altered at least once during the eight weeks preceding the start of the clinical trial, which meant that they were not eligible for the study. However, they were still entered – but the case report forms for these patients stated that their treatment had not altered during the preceding eight weeks.

- Although the hospital outpatient register confirmed the appointments for the patients in the study for their first and fourth visits, the register showed no appointments for them on the reported dates of their second and third visits.
- Some of the ECG tracings and some of the patients' x rays had been cut to remove either the date on which they were taken, or the patient identification, or both.
- There was no evidence in certain cases that x rays were ever taken at all.
- A number of patients were purported to have been seen on three separate Scottish Bank Holidays when the hospital outpatient department was closed.
- Thirteen patient visits were purported to have taken place when Dr Anderton was on holiday, but there was no evidence of recorded cover during this period.
- Compared with the results reported from other centres taking part in the second study, which was reviewed by the company, Dr Anderton's results showed remarkable consistency in the intervals between patient visits, and in the timing of taking blood samples. On the other hand, he demonstrated a rise in blood drug metabolite levels when every other centre demonstrated a fall, he reported one-eighth of the adverse events per patient reported by the other centres – those adverse events, which he did report, being exactly as indicated on the data sheet for the products in question, whereas many of the other reported adverse events differed widely from those included in the data sheet.

The case was submitted to the General Medical Council and, at the hearing of the professional conduct committee, Dr Anderton pleaded guilty to a charge of serious professional misconduct. Despite receiving a number of character references from some of his distinguished colleagues, the committee directed that his name be erased from the Medical Register.

The case of the unstressed rats

In January 1994 the head of a British university department of psychology wrote to a pharmaceutical company in France suggesting that a research project be conducted in his department on the effects of an investigational drug in a realistic animal model of stress. Following consideration of this letter, the company drafted an agreement between itself and the professor, taking into account that the professor had developed an animal model inducing chronic mild stress in the rat and that the company was interested in the testing of a new medicine for the treatment of stress. For performing this study the professor's department was to be paid an agreed sum of money.

The member of staff who was designated by the professor to conduct this study was a postgraduate student in psychology, who was interested in the animal model that was to be used for this study. Her own experimental findings, however, led her to conclude that, whereas the drinking of sucrose solution was said to be reduced when rats were subjected to a battery of mild stresses, the drinking of sucrose solution was significantly *increased* when the rats were further stressed. After subsequent discussion with the professor she repeated her experiment using, first, outbred rats – with the same result – and then with inbred rats. The experiment with these last rats demonstrated a transient reduction in sucrose drinking after mild stress, but this returned to normal after three weeks, and after two further weeks the stressed rats increased their sucrose drinking just as the rats in her two previous experiments had done.

When she conducted the experiment with the rats yet again, she found no difference in sucrose drinking at all between the two groups. She sought to find a reason why her experimental findings failed to match the model and came up with a possible explanation. Regardless of this, however, the professor ordered the student to repeat the study with the control rats becoming the experimental rats and vice versa. On this occasion there was a reduction in sucrose drinking in the rats which had previously been the controls – but as there were, in effect, now no controls, the observation was considered meaningless. Nevertheless she was further instructed to begin treatment with the investigational drug but this made no observable difference to the drinking patterns of either groups of rats.

Her conclusions were that:

- the differences observed between the results she obtained in her experiments and those described by the professor in his original papers were profound, suggesting that the chronic mild stress model was flawed;
- the switch between controls and experimental rats in the repeat experiment rendered that experiment invalid;
- there was no evidence that the investigational drug effected any changes in the experimental rats.

The case was submitted to MedicoLegal Investigations and a detailed comparison was made between the reports submitted to the company by the professor in December 1994 and April 1996 with the data yielded by the postgraduate student when she conducted the study herself, and a number of differences were noted:

- Inappropriate sucrose data appear to have been used and analysed.
- Critical sucrose data have been omitted.
- The fact that an effect, which had disappeared by week 2, was hidden.
- Experimental groups were not matched.
- So-called drug-induced differences were likely to be the result of differences between groups that existed before the drug was administered.
- Inappropriate mean sucrose intake values (and standard errors of the mean) were used.
- Values were inserted for missing values from the original data set without justification.

- Inappropriate statistical analyses were used and the significant results presented could not be replicated.
- The fact that the groups had been switched – thus rendering the study invalid – was not mentioned.

The inconsistencies and anomalies revealed in this case could not be accounted for by pure chance, nor were they satisfactorily explained. There was therefore what appeared to be *prima facie* evidence of the generation of false data with an intention to deceive, amounting to serious professional misconduct, which justified referral to the Vice-Chancellor of the university concerned. The outcome of the handling of this case by the university was far from satisfactory, but the professor is no longer in post.

The case of the eminent St Helens GP

The case of Dr Geoffrey Fairhurst, an eminent general practitioner in St Helens, Lancashire is discussed fully in Chapters 15 and 16. On this occasion it was the doctor's partner who acted as whistleblower and who alerted the authorities to activities which Fairhurst was clearly doing his best to conceal.[14]

Conclusion

The above cases, and others, came from a variety of sources – astute clinical trial monitors and quality assurance professionals supported by their companies, and whistleblowers from amongst research nurses, partners in general practice, research ethics committees, health authorities, a PhD student, and a disillusioned pharmaceutical physician. The important lesson to remember is that suspicion demands investigation, either to stop the misconduct, particularly where it involves the exploitation of patients, or to establish that no misconduct exists – both with the minimum of delay. A practical policy, which has been adopted by the industry and slowly adapted and introduced within universities and health authorities, is as follows:

1 Every pharmaceutical company should be reminded of its obligations under the principles of Good Clinical (Research) Practice, and asked to state its commitment to reporting all cases of fraud and to taking appropriate action.
2 Every company, university and health authority should introduce Standard Operating Procedures for the handling of suspected research misconduct, which should include at least the following items:
   a. A clear statement of policy towards the handling of suspected data.
   b. A stated policy that any cause for concern regarding suspected research misconduct must be referred to the medical director (or other specified appropriate person) at the earliest possible stage.

c. Clear guidelines as to the path to be followed once fraud is suspected.

d. Clear guidelines as to the right of appeal if a complainant feels that his/her concern is being inappropriately addressed.

e. Access to appropriate statistical screening methods which can be used efficiently on a routine basis.

f. A policy that all cases involving clinical trials on medicinal products, which give rise to serious concern regarding a specific investigator, should be notified at an early stage to the ABPI Director of Medical Affairs.

Clearly it is important that anyone involved in the detection of suspected research misconduct needs advice and guidance, given that, in spite of the thrust of this book, a suspicion of research misconduct will remain a rare event. Advice on where such guidance is available can come from the ABPI, which is absolutely committed to giving all possible assistance in advising on action against fraud. Appropriate publicity should be given to the outcome of such action, to act as a deterrent, in a determination to minimise fraud and misconduct in clinical research. Only the utmost vigour in applying this policy will be successful; it is in the ultimate interests of patient safety to do so. Would that official bodies recognised these priorities as well.

References

1 *Declaration of Helsinki* (amended 1975, 1983, 1989, 1996, 2000). Ferney-Voltaire, France: World Medical Association, 2000.
2 Campbell D. Medicine needs its MI5. *BMJ* 1997;**315**:1677–80.
3 European Union Note for Guidance. *Good clinical practice for trials on medicinal products.* Brussels: European Commission, 1991.
4 International Conference on Harmonisation. *Good clinical practices.* Geneva: International Federation of Pharmaceutical Manufacturing Associations, 1996.
5 Lock SP. Resumé of recent events. In: *Fraud and misconduct in medical research*, Second edition. London: BMJ Books, 1996.
6 Anonymous. GMC professional conduct committee. *BMJ* 1988;**296**:306.
7 Royal College of Physicians of London. *Report on fraud and misconduct in medical research.* London: Royal College of Physicians, 1991.
8 Wells F. Fraud and misconduct in clinical research. In: Griffin J, O'Grady J, Wells F, eds. *The textbook of pharmaceutical medicine.* Belfast: Queens University, 1994.
9 *Proceedings of the Royal College of Physicians of Edinburgh* (Suppl.) January 2000.
10 Dyer O. GMC finds GPs guilty of fraud. *BMJ* 1994;**308**:1122.
11 Dyer O. GP found guilty of forging trial consent forms. *BMJ* 1998;**317**:1475.
12 Gillespie F, Reynolds M. GP in huge fraud probe. *Cambridge Evening News* 10 December 1997.
13 Mitchell P. Edinburgh doctor struck off because of clinical-trial fraud. *Lancet* 1997;**350**:272.
14 Dyer O. GP struck off for fraud in drug trials. *BMJ* 1996;**312**:798.

PART III
NATIONAL PRACTICAL ISSUES

6: A pharmaceutical company's approach to the threat of research fraud

PETER BROCK

The increased concern since 1990 about fraud in pharmaceutical industry-sponsored research has been criticised by many people as being a gross overreaction to a minor problem, but the emphasis on fraud occurring in *clinical* research is a greater concern.

Clinical research is almost at the end of the research and development chain for a pharmaceutical product. Very many important decisions are made much earlier on the basis of one or two critical experiments. Often dosage recommendations for initial clinical work are based on pharmacokinetic data derived from a small number of animals, and often the results are not duplicated. The carcinogenic risk or toxic risk to humans is often extrapolated from one or two pivotal toxicology studies. On the other hand it is very unlikely that key decisions concerning the assessment of risk or dosage would be based on a single clinical comparative trial.

Thus, unreliable data, particularly in relation to toxicology or pharmacology, could have much more serious implications than fraud occurring in a single phase III or phase IV clinical study. Companies should therefore be equally vigilant with regard to preclinical experiments as to clinical experiments in humans. Unfortunately, from the general public's perspective, this does not seem to have been the case.

Many of the earlier cases of fraud that have been drawn to the public's attention have been relatively trivial examples occurring in postmarketing surveillance or large scale general practice studies. More recently, however, cases of fraud in earlier phase research have come to public notice. The relative importance of early phase research must commit a company to having the most stringent checks and balances to ensure that all data coming out of early phase research are genuine and validated.

Despite the concern that undue emphasis has been placed on clinical research, as distinct from early phase research, most of the steps that companies are introducing to protect themselves against clinical research fraud are equally applicable to in-house or contract research.

In this chapter I will outline some of the approaches that can be adopted by companies in order to protect themselves against clinical fraud, because that is where most experience has been obtained.

Why commit fraud?

A thorough knowledge of the motivation to commit fraud could provide companies with a permanent cure to the problem. Unfortunately such a panacea does not exist but some of the factors that motivate investigators to commit fraud are obvious and well documented.

Peer pressure

There have been numerous examples, mainly in academic research, of peer pressure leading to the need to publish a continuous stream of articles or to achieve "a breakthrough" in a particular topic. This is well documented but there seems little that can be done to ameliorate this academic peer group pressure.

Unreasonable expectations

The industry, in its constant drive to shorten the development time for new pharmaceuticals, exerts considerable pressure on its research and discovery group. Simple calculations can show that each month's delay in product licence approval, in a major country, can lead to loss of sales revenue of many millions of pounds. In the light of this pressure it is not surprising that there have been cases where short cuts have been taken in the development process. Sometimes these short cuts have led to the fraudulent generation of data.

An investigator, with a proven track record in a fairly simple and straightforward study, is asked by the company to do a second or third study. The new study, however, is a much more complex design, much more stretching scientifically, and requires much more commitment both of time and effort from the investigator. The investigator feels embarrassed to admit that he does not properly understand the study, the company assumes because he has done the earlier study well that he is "a good investigator", and does not take the time adequately to explain what is required of him. This is a recipe for disaster.

Greed

It is, however, a sad reflection on the standards of some investigators that the only motivation that can be identified for their committing forgery or fraud is straightforward greed. Many acts of fraud in clinical research have been linked to trivial studies involving small sums of money. It is therefore difficult to understand how greed could be a motivating factor. Further analysis does, however, show that quite often the company has conveyed the idea that these studies are trivial (occasionally postmarketing surveillance is the culprit here) and this has communicated itself to the investigator. The unscrupulous investigator feels, therefore, that as the study is trivial he will treat it trivially and has a licence to defraud.

It is obvious that company culture, approach, and attitude, or academia's approach and attitude, are common factors. In tackling the problem of fraud, it therefore seems that a change in attitude on behalf of the company or academia should be the key to success.

Who commits fraud?

The distressing answer to this question is that all layers of company organisations, from external investigators through trial monitors, people engaged in data resolution, data processing, and project management, to medical directors, have all at one time or another been involved in allegations of clinical fraud.

This observation is very important for companies aiming to eradicate fraud from their research process. It means that companies must have systems that allow suspicion and checking of all levels of the organisation up to and including senior management. This is hard to achieve in practice.

The prime aim of every company must be to build in checks and balances that allow appeal to "a higher authority", if a complainant feels that his or her immediate line manager is not responding appropriately to the complaint.

The company's dilemma: between a rock and a hard place

If we conclude that a change in attitude on behalf of the company or academic department could be a key to success in combating fraud the obvious question to ask is "Why hasn't this happened before?"

To understand why the pharmaceutical industry has been loath, until relatively recently, to tackle the problem of fraud, one has to understand the unique relationship that exists between the pharmaceutical industry and its customers.

In the normal relationship of a company carrying out a process, a supplier of goods, and an end user or customer, the supplier supplies the raw material, which is then processed by the manufacturer and sold to a customer. The transactions are one way. In this scheme the customer can impose standards on the manufacturer and the manufacturer can impose standards on his supplier.

The situation that the pharmaceutical industry finds itself in with regard to clinical research is that our suppliers – in this case clinicians – are normally our customers, prescribing doctors. This has been one of the prime reasons why the pharmaceutical industry has been loath to take an aggressive attitude to clinical fraud.

A case study might make the problem clear.

The case of Dr X

The clinical research department of a large pharmaceutical company carried out a large postmarketing surveillance study on its new cardiovascular agent. In the routine screening of the data, suspicion was raised that a certain doctor, Doctor X, had fraudulently generated the data. A site visit was initiated and the site monitor confirmed that it was highly likely that Doctor X had committed fraud.

After documentation of the case, it was drawn to the attention of the medical director, who decided to pursue the doctor for fraud. As was the company's custom, the medical director's intention to prosecute the case was drawn to the attention of the marketing and sales directors and the chief executive officer.

Three days after the joint staff meeting to discuss the case, a note was received from the national sales manager concerning Doctor X. The note read:

Doctor X is one of the best doctors that we have in the country for prescribing our whole range of products. Our local representative confirms that Doctor X is a "company friend" and any prosecution brought against Doctor X would have a major impact on our sales in that area. Not only is Doctor X a keen user of the company products but he has been used extensively to speak at local and regional meetings in support of our products particularly in light of his first hand knowledge of their use.

I therefore recommend to the CEO that no further action be taken against Doctor X despite the fact that the case seems proven against him.

The commercial decision not to prosecute Doctor X was upheld by the chief executive officer and no further action was taken. This, however, is not the end of the saga.

Unbeknown to the sales and marketing directors, the medical director had asked the research group to check their computer database to see if Doctor X had participated in other studies. Two or three days later it was confirmed that Doctor X had participated in at least two other studies and one large postmarketing surveillance exercise. The data were retrieved from these studies and checked, and a high index of suspicion that fraud had been committed in these studies was confirmed.

In addition the national sales manager, presumably out of interest, had been checking the representative call statistics to see how often Doctor X had been called on by the local representative. He was amazed to find that for the past two years Doctor X had been seen between 10 and 16 times a year despite the fact that the maximum call frequency allowed within the company was four to six calls a year even on high users of company products.

At this stage several people were getting extremely concerned and it was decided to check, through independent audit, whether Doctor X was in fact a high user of company products as he had claimed. *As far as could be told from an in-depth audit using third party sources, Doctor X was in fact not a user of company products at all.*

The myth therefore of the "company friend", the good doctor whom we do not want to upset, was in this case exploded. It was, however, serendipity that the investigation of Doctor X was carried further because of the interest of the medical director and the national sales manager. It is a salutory note that, despite the additional information, no further action was taken against Doctor X.

Not only was Doctor X defrauding the clinical research department, he was in fact defrauding the representatives and the company – particularly when it is borne in mind that the company was using him, and paying an honorarium, to speak about his first hand knowledge of company products to other doctors.

The dilemma posed by the unique relationship with the customer as the supplier, and the need to protect company friends, as illustrated by this case, is still a major hurdle to the industry's commitment to stamping out fraud in clinical research.

The position in the United Kingdom since 1989 has improved considerably. The positive approach taken by the Association of the British Pharmaceutical Industry and the very firm line taken by the General Medical Council (GMC) have reinforced the British pharmaceutical industry's decision to eradicate fraud from clinical research. The GMC in its 1992 annual report made the following comment:

The Council is bound to take a serious view of behaviour such as that outlined above [proved clinical fraud], in relation to clinical trials. Lack of care or dishonesty by doctors when participating in such trials is not only discreditable in itself, but is also a potential source of danger to patients, whose safety depends on the integrity and diligence of all those who participate in the testing of approved drugs.

This unambiguous statement has proved very helpful ever since in convincing companies and organisations to adopt an aggressive approach to suspected fraud.

Prevention or cure

The old adage that prevention is better than cure applies to fraud in clinical research. The cost, inconvenience, and delays incurred by having to redo clinical studies because of lack of confidence in data obtained from a pivotal research project are enormous. Although this chapter will review some of the methods that have been used to detect fraud once it has been committed, the aim of a company should be to prevent fraud being perpetrated against it, not to detect when fraud has been committed. In fact the detection of a fraud perpetrated against a company should be seen as a failure of the company systems, and just as much a criticism of the company as of the person committing the crime.

In a company's attempt to prevent fraud, its attitude and that of its employees is of prime importance. A full and frank discussion covering the company's approach to fraud and its methods used to detect it can act as a major deterrent to an investigator tempted to take short cuts with the study. To achieve this, trial monitors, clinical research associates, medical advisers, and all other people having contact with investigators must have adequate training to make sure that the right message is communicated. A company that gives the impression that a research project is "trivial" cannot expect it to be taken seriously by an investigator.

The application of the guidelines on good clinical practice and good clinical research practice[1-3] with the checks and balances they introduce, and the structured approach to the writing of protocol, design of case record forms, and archiving of documentation, have done much to convince investigators that clinical research is a serious issue for the pharmaceutical industry. This change in attitude, and the benefits that come with it, should be one of the main reasons for applying good clinical research practice to all phases of clinical research, not just studies being done for regulatory purposes.

A way to further emphasise the company's insistence on reliable and accurate data is to have a formal contract between the investigator and the company. This is often called "The investigator agreement". This contract, as well as covering finance, timing, etc., should include the following items:

- a statement that the research is to be carried out according to the good clinical practice guidelines (GCP) (If necessary a brief guide to these could be attached to make sure that there was no uncertainty about what this meant);
- a statement that the company reserves the right to audit or do source data verification in order to check the accuracy of the data;
- a statement that it is company policy to pursue all cases of suspected clinical fraud according to a standard operating procedure; if the standard operating procedure is attached, the potential investigator is left in no doubt as to the consequences of fraud.

The role of the standard operating procedure

With the introduction of good clinical research practice, standard operating procedures now govern all aspects of clinical research. Every company should have a standard operating procedure outlining what is required of its employees in cases of suspected fraud.

Such a standard operating procedure achieves two objectives. Firstly, it can be used to show would-be investigators the company's approach to fraud and thus convince them of the seriousness with which this is viewed by the company. Secondly, it offers some protection, at least in English law, for people who act according to the standard operating procedure, who may be threatened with litigation by persons suspected of committing fraud. This is particularly important in those cases where, on further investigation according to the processes laid out in the standard operating procedure, the suspicion is found to be unfounded.

In order for the limited protection offered by such a standard operating procedure to be maximised, it should clearly and unequivocally state the exact process that should be adopted by someone who has a suspicion that clinical fraud has taken place. It should be unequivocal and allow no deviation from the steps outlined. Further protection can be obtained if the job descriptions of those engaged in clinical research state that compliance with the standard operating procedures currently in force (including the one on fraud) is a requirement for employment.

As well as offering the benefits outlined above, a company standard operating procedure, if properly written, can offer the right advice and guidance to junior staff who have reason to use this procedure, which, we hope, is only rarely called on. The junior clinical research associate who is suspicious of the world-famous professor at a time when all her senior colleagues are on holiday would find a clearly written standard operating procedure of tremendous use.

An example of a standard operating procedure is given in Appendix A.

Detecting clinical fraud

The detection of clinical fraud is not easy. Some formal scheme is necessary particularly if approaches to the problem are going to be carried forward into a training programme. A scheme that has been found to work well in practice is to consider the detection of fraud in four distinct steps:

1 The visit, normally by clinical research associate, medical research associate, or medical adviser
2 The return trial materials
3 The case record forms, patient diary cards, etc.
4 The final report.

The visit

For companies that have fully implemented GCP into everyday working, initiation visits are required before the setting up of a clinical trial. These visits provide the ideal opportunity to assess the reliability, effectiveness, and, sometimes, honesty of the centres being considered to participate in a research programme.

To fully exploit the opportunity presented by these early visits and the planning of clinical research a certain approach is necessary from the company representative. Many company representatives (clinical research associates or medical research associates) involved in the initiation visits for clinical research are new graduates in their first professional post. They need to understand that, if they have the slightest concern that something is not right with the centre or the investigator, this should be communicated to the responsible person in the company. Many new graduates find this very difficult to put into practice, particularly if dealing with well-known or prestigious investigators or centres. Strong reassurance from their management on the importance of this issue is needed.

95

In helping clinical research staff to identify the "giveaway signs" conveyed during a study initiation visit, training and the sharing of experience are the keys to success. With encouragement, trial monitors will rapidly build up a bibliography of relevant quotes or situations or attitudes that may indicate a possible future problem.

Some noteworthy quotes

"I won't actually be doing the work, my ... will be, but you can't meet them today because they are off somewhere else."

(At a study or site initiation visit): "I'll be getting the patients from several other clinics/outpatients, but I am not quite sure which ones I will use yet, I will let you know."

(At a monitoring visit): "I don't have the patient's records here, but if you know what the questions are, I will follow them up and send the answers to you."

It is common practice, in fact some people would say the norm, for the principal investigator not to be the person who will actually do the work. Under these conditions it is essential that the company be given access to the staff who will be ultimately responsible for carrying out the studies. It is all too easy for a prestigious or busy unit to take on more and more work in the hope, without checking, that the junior staff can cope with it. Under these conditions unreasonable pressures are brought to bear on junior staff, fearful for their future, to complete the studies.

To illustrate some of the problems a further case study is useful.

The case of study A

A British based pharmaceutical company was preparing to do a pivotal pharmacokinetic study on a new clinical lead. The study was aimed at establishing the pharmacokinetics of the new product in an elderly population.

The company had not carried out pharmacokinetic studies in elderly patients in the United Kingdom before and so had problems in selecting a suitable centre. A literature search was carried out and a centre was chosen on the basis of published work. The centre was visited by the clinical projects manager concerned to check that it was capable of doing the study according to the company's standard operating procedures.

At this visit the project manager spoke with the head of department, who reassured him by reference to previous work, both published and unpublished, and a review of the documentation from previous studies that the unit was equipped and able to do the work required. The principal investigator emphasised that the work would be carried out in a six-bedded unit which was an offshoot, separate from the main ward of another hospital. A protocol was developed, based on a protocol provided by the parent company and all the appropriate signatures were obtained.

At this time the medical director of the company was asked to sign the protocol but remembered the investigator's name from previous conversations with colleagues at a pharmaceutical function a few weeks before. On checking up with his colleagues he found that the centre had an unreliable track record over the past six months or so, but had been a reliable unit before that. The medical director refused to sign the protocol and instructed the project manager to return to the unit to confirm that it was suitable and able to do the work required.

On this occasion the project manager made an appointment to visit the unit concerned, although this was difficult. On arrival he was greeted by a rather harassed registrar, who explained that the "unit" was in fact a curtained off area in one of the main geriatric wards and was currently full of routine admissions because of a flu epidemic. The junior staff member also confirmed that there was a backlog of studies waiting in the unit but staff cuts over the past six months, owing to hospital cutbacks, had made it more and more difficult to carry out the work.

Needless to say the study never actually went ahead but it is problematical whether it would ever have been completed or, more importantly, whether, if it had apparently been completed, it would have been done fraudulently.

Sometimes visits by clinical research associates can produce unexpected results:

The case of trial P: the unusual consequences of monitoring visits by clinical research associates

A large multicentre study of an injectable anti-infective agent for the management of intra-abdominal sepsis was being carried out by a European-based company. Monitoring visits by the clinical research associate were, after the initiation and set-up visits, to be held at monthly intervals.

One particular centre caught the attention of the data administrator, who plotted out the recruitment rate for the suspicious centre and all other centres.

This showed that at the end of month two, after the clinical research associates had been on a motivational campaign, recruitment picked up from five per month to just about six per month for most centres and then returned down to the baseline recruitment rate of five per month until the visit at the end of month five. At this point the clinical research associates told the investigators that recruitment was closing in one month with the inevitable upswing in recruitment rate.

With the suspect centre the upswing in recruitment after the visit at the end of month two was a little above average but not suspicious. What was suspicious was the very dramatic (in fact in this case doubling) increase of recruitment of patients when the investigator was informed that the study would close for recruitment in one or two months' time and no further patients would qualify for payment. Further investigation revealed that at least four of the patients recruited after the visit at the end of month four were not included in the study.

Monitoring for patterns or trends in documentation that may raise suspicion

Historically, clinical research was often analysed with the use of accounting paper, pencil, and rubber. The volumes of data collected were limited and it was possible to look at complete data sets and get a very good "feel for the data". Many experienced statisticians still insist on obtaining this "feel for the data" before subjecting them to statistical analysis.

The introduction of modern computer methods has to a large measure removed manual manipulation of the data. The need to process case record forms as if they are items on a production line, to avoid peaks and troughs of workload in the data group, has exacerbated the problem. Monitoring visits by field staff are often spaced out over many weeks or months, and case record forms will have moved on to the next level within the data processing organisation.

The first suspicion of fraud is often on a "gut feeling" of primary or secondary monitors. In order to encourage this intuitive approach, it is often useful to reacquire all the case record forms relating to a particular doctor or centre and to review them all together. This is particularly the case if there are other grounds for suspicion. This longitudinal review of the data, all in one place and at one time, may draw attention to suspicious similarities that have been missed when individual case record forms have been handled on a one by one basis as they move through the system.

There are many giveaway signs, too many to list here, that may point to forgery or fraud. In one example the use of a distinctive green colour ink to complete the case record forms on approximately 60 patients from three different centres over a six month period was suspicious. Patient diary cards, particularly those requiring the patients to enter data and symptoms or complete questionnaires or visual analogue scales, can be particularly revealing. Similarities in handwriting between "patients" or the way that the "patient" has marked the visual analogue line can often be the clue that initiates a fraud investigation.

Of particular interest is the wide variety of ways that patients choose to mark visual analogue lines if given a free choice, as they normally are; the use of a cross, tick, oblique or horizontal line, or even a bar commencing at one end of the visual analogue scale and finishing at the patient's preferred point will all be seen. Lack of this variability in patient's completed visual analogue scales allegedly coming from different patients should be viewed with great suspicion.

The dating game

Many cases of fraud are committed without much thought on the part of the person perpetrating the crime. Often the fraud is committed in a great hurry, particularly if the motivation is to complete the work by an agreed deadline. Under these circumstances quite obvious and silly mistakes are made. The person committing the crime is often more concerned to check that the follow ups actually occur 10, 14, 28, or 60 days – whatever the protocol dictates – after the previous visit than to ensure that these dates actually fall on days of the week that make sense. It is not unusual to find that some investigators seem to be doing a lot of clinics on a Sunday and even routine follow up outpatient endoscopies on Christmas Day have occasionally been noted. In one dramatic example a whole cohort of patients were claimed to have been followed up at a time when it was known that the unit was shut for refurbishment.

The trial materials

The clinical practice requires that all unused trial materials be accounted for on completion of a clinical study.

Of all the aspects that clinical trial monitors and clinical research associates find most fascinating, the one that captures the imagination is the review or audit of returned clinical trial materials. Quite often the first hint of trouble occurs after the review of returned trial materials.

It pays to be suspicious – bearing in mind that trial materials normally have been in a patient's home, handbag, pocket, or kitchen cabinet – if they seem to be too clean, too exact, or too similar. From my experience, trial materials that are actually taken as prescribed are very suspicious indeed. Although it is generally accepted that compliance in clinical trials is higher than compliance in routine medical practice, materials taken exactly as dispensed should be viewed with a great deal of scepticism.

The widespread introduction of calendar packing and blister packing has also provided a fruitful area for investigation. Calendar packs which start on the same day are obviously worthy of investigation. It is sometimes particularly illuminating to check the day of the week that it seems the medication was started on against the start date as entered on the case record form.

One of the mainstays of the detection of fraud is the recognition that a person's habitual behaviour will be reflected in the case record forms or other activities associated with the study. The use of blister packaging has led to some interesting examples. In one particular study of an antidepressant, it seems that the medication was being taken properly but examination of returned blister packages from several different "patients" showed that they had all started their medication from the same physical location on the blister strip. Obviously this is very unlikely to occur in real practice.

Two more case studies will further illustrate possible approaches in reviewing returned trial materials.

The case of trial Z

Trial Z was a study with a topical application (gel formulation) of a non-steroidal anti-inflammatory drug carried out in the United Kingdom. It was a parallel group, multicentre, double blind placebo-controlled study using 20 centres, with 12 patients per centre.

At the first follow up visit to one particular centre, when the first two to three patients entered a review, the trial monitor voiced some concerns suggesting possible fraud. The monitor had noted that the returned trial materials all seemed to have been handled the same way. The tubes had been squeezed in an identical fashion. The monitor commented, "There are four people living in our house, we all squeeze our toothpaste differently – how is it that the three patients enrolled into the study at this centre seem to have squeezed their tubes identically – not only that, but the tubes seem to have been gripped in the middle and squeezed, very unlikely for a medication that was meant to have been given three to four times a day for five to seven days." At a subsequent visit the remaining tubes for the last nine patients from that centre all looked identical.

The returned samples for this centre were also unique in that their weights were a mean of $24\,g \pm 6\,g$, whereas the tubes returned from the other centres showed a mean weight of $8\,g \pm 12\,g$. Examination of all the tubes returned from the suspect centre showed that they had all been gripped and squeezed in an identical manner – making it very unlikely that the materials had been used in the clinical trial by 12 different patients.

The case of trial Y

Trial Y was a study of an oral non-steroidal anti-inflammatory drug. It was a prospective, double blind, placebo-controlled, crossover study carried out as part of a phase III programme. Escape analgesia (paracetamol) was provided. The consumption rates for the escape analgesia were calculated on a daily basis and were one of the parameters of efficacy.

The centre carrying out the study had a proven track record in similar work and seemed to have carried out previous studies quickly and efficiently.

The company statistician was the first to point out an anomaly. It was obvious from reviewing the data that, in those treatment periods when the patients should have been receiving the active drug, their analgesic consumption seemed to remain the same as when they were receiving placebo. As previous studies had shown efficacy this was very suspicious.

There were three explanations: there had been problems in clinical trial materials – not unknown – and the active drug was in fact missing from the treatment schedules (that is, the patients received placebo all the time); or, secondly, the drug was not active; or, thirdly, the patients were not taking the medication.

Analysis of retention samples, or surplus materials unallocated from the trial programme, and of returned samples from the study, confirmed that the active drug was present in the appropriate tablets. A review of the blister packaging of the trial materials suggested that the patients were in fact taking them as directed. A review of other clinical trial data suggested that the dose being given in this study was adequate to achieve an analgesic effect, which should have led to a reduction in the consumption of escape analgesia.

Audit confirmed that the patients actually existed but there was no evidence that they had participated in the clinical study (this study was carried out before GCP was widely introduced in the United Kingdom). Subsequently the investigator admitted that he had made up all the data and had disposed of the escape analgesia leaving "just a few" tablets in the bottle.

Routine examination of the data: a time consuming exercise

Once data have been loaded into a database, particularly with online computer systems, which are now widely available, it becomes simplicity itself to carry out comprehensive analysis of data sets. This can be a useful exercise and Chapter 14 by Evans gives details of the principles behind such analysis and the various methods available. Many companies have introduced the routine review of data by such methods as part of their quality assurance procedures.

Interpretation of data derived from such comparisons should, however, be undertaken with extreme care. I have known several cases where suspicion was raised by the "atypical" nature of the data from a centre. Further investigation revealed, however, that the data were quite genuine and the difference was due to either an unusual age/sex distribution within that centre or particular referral patterns happening within a hospital or community. It is therefore, I think, unwise to base any case of suspected fraud simply on this sort of analysis.

The returned case record forms

Case record forms are used and completed in a working environment. A data monitor from a major international company once said at a meeting that, "The case record form returned without at least four coffee stains and four different pens used in its completion has invariably been fraudulently filled in." This is probably an extreme view, but case record forms which are returned too quickly, too clean, too complete (with no data resolutions), and too uniform, in terms of both the style of handwriting and pens used, should be viewed with considerable suspicion.

Having given some indication of the methods that can be used for detecting fraudulent centres, I must emphasise that by far the bigger problem is the detection of a single fraudulent entry, or series of entries, relating to a particular patient within a centre or to a particular visit. A missing value may be fraudulently completed when all other data are complete and when company employees are placed under excessive pressure to complete a study. Under other conditions, fraud occasionally occurs if a particular patient, whose record is complete in all other respects, misses a follow up appointment for any reason; the data for the missed visits are then invented. The detection of this type of fraud is incredibly difficult.

If the investigator, or company employee, has inserted clinically sensible values, taking into account an individual patient's previous and subsequent results, a fraud may be impossible to detect without source data verification.

The study report

Speculation continues as to whether fraud is ever detected by the time the final report is written. This has actually occurred but such cases seem to be few and far between. Quite often the observations that lead to the detection of fraud in a clinical report are serendipitous.

The cases of companies D and F

Two medical directors of major international companies were discussing, over a gin and tonic, the cost of clinical pharmacology in contract research establishments in the UK. As is often the case, both were talking from recent examples and the conversation progressed to discussion of the design of the studies.

It became obvious to the two directors that they were talking about almost identical studies, being carried out at the same contract house, with similar agents. Both of these were cardiovascular agents potentially useful in treating hypertension.

As the evening wore on, it became obvious not only that they were talking about a similar study design with similar agents but that the results that they had obtained in their studies were similar if not identical. The two directors agreed, far into the night, to exchange final reports; they were not suspicious that any of the data had been fraudulently generated at this time.

At a subsequent meeting they compared notes because, when the reports were read, it was impossible to detect the difference between them other than that the name of the molecule had been changed. Even the shapes of the kinetic curves were identical and the calculated clearances and half lives were very similar.

To this date neither of the medical directors knows whether the data had been fraudulently generated. Needless to say both reports were abandoned, at substantial cost, both in terms of money paid to the centre and of delay in getting product licence approval.

The value of source data verification audit as a method for detecting research fraud

In theory 100% audit with source data verification should lead to a 100% detection of research fraud. In practice 100% audit is impossible within the bounds of reasonable costs. Most companies therefore have decided to introduce sampling methods, which by definition guarantee less than 100% verification.

At the present rate of development in the UK of source data verification, it cannot be relied on to detect all cases of clinical fraud. As the methods develop and GCP and source data verification become the accepted norm, it will undoubtedly be harder for clinical fraud to be committed in British research.

It is also particularly difficult, in the UK, to use all the information derived from source data verification audit in the prosecution of a case of suspected fraud. Quite often an audit report might contain a phrase as follows:

Careful inspection of the case notes showed that many (16/24) visited the surgery during the trial period for either flu vaccination, blood pressure checks, or for routine examination or follow up for prescriptions. Dr Y commented that the record keeping is not as complete as it should be but that this was a general practice surgery not a research organisation.

Many sets of case notes had a separate new "support card" filled in with the same pen and handwriting. Dr W commented that those who did not have a separate card were seen at home.

There are some doubtful details recorded in the notes, where, for example, some statements have been deleted and then written over with a different pen.

The role of ethics committees

A good case can be made for ethics committees to have a pivotal role in the prevention, detection and management of suspected fraud and Chapter 13 by Blunt covers this in more detail. The requirement for ethics committees to be aware of the ICH GCP guidelines will be more readily appreciated once the EC directive on clinical trials is adopted. Meanwhile, at least in the UK, this challenge clearly seems to have been picked up by local research ethics committees.

Where a protocol is submitted to a local research ethics committee for its consideration along with the name of the proposed investigator and centre, and the committee has doubts that the doctor could recruit the number of patients required by the protocol, or perhaps has some concerns about the quality of work previously carried out by the centre or doctor, then it is ethically reasonable for it to draw this to the attention of the company before the initiation of the clinical study.

What should the pharmaceutical industry do about it?

The way forward for the pharmaceutical industry seems clear. To avoid clinical fraud being perpetrated the following process should be introduced and built into the control of the clinical research:

- The full implementation of GCP for all clinical studies
- The setting up of an investigator contract, signed by both investigator and company, which outlines the responsibilities of the investigator and

103

company and specifies what action the company will take if it suspects fraud has been perpetrated against it

- A declaration that the company is willing to prosecute all cases of fraud
- The training of clinical research associates, trial monitors, data managers, and medical advisers to be alert to the telltale signs of fraud
- The building in of routine check statistics to the analysis of data
- The introduction of a standard operating procedure, signed by all levels of management, both commercial and clinical, which outlines unambiguously the steps to be followed in cases of suspected clinical fraud.

The next major step forward must be the generation and sharing of details of cases of suspected fraud among companies, the trade associations, and the boards of health and ethics committees. This, sadly, remains something for the future but how good it would be if it came to pass.

References

1 Harvard Medical School. *Guidelines for investigators in scientific research.* Cambridge, Mass: Office of the Dean for Academic Affairs, 1988.
2 Association of the British Pharmaceutical Industry. *Good clinical research practice guidelines.* London: ABPI, 1988.
3 Committee on Proprietary Medicinal Products Working Party on Efficacy of Medicinal Products. *Good clinical practice for trials on medicinal products in the European Community.* [111 3976/88-EN Final.] Brussels: European Commission, 1991.

7: Role of the FDA, NIH, and other bodies in the United States

ARTHUR HOROWITZ

During the past several years, we have witnessed a dramatic change in the clinical trial landscape. These changes have included more clinical studies (more clinical investigators and sites per study); expansion and fluidity of the clinical investigator pool; new players in new parts; and new technologies. The rush to market a new drug and competition among newly acquired large multinational companies have created increased pressures on cost and time. Each year, there are more original New Drug Applications resulting in new product competition. In 1999, $5.79 billion US dollars were spent by the Pharmaceutical Research Manufacturers Association (PhRMA) member companies in Phase I–III activities. The average daily cost of delay in market introduction is estimated to be $1.3 million US dollars.[1] To avoid delay and to improve efficiency in a shortage of company capacity and talent, companies are outsourcing to more contract research organisations and site management organisations as well as hiring more clinical investigators.

The number of new clinical investigators conducting one trial has increased 30% annually during the past four years (Figure 7.1). An

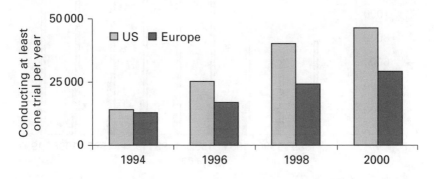

Figure 7.1   Proliferation of clinical investigators. (Source: CenterWatch)

increasing number of clinical researchers are private clinicians not associated with academia, where the desire to participate in clinical research is driven by the desire for more knowledge or career advancement. The number of private doctors in research has almost tripled as illustrated in Figure 7.2. It has become a multibillion dollar industry, with drug companies working with thousands of private doctors. In this era of managed care, at any rate, in the USA, companies are urging private doctors to join the lucrative clinical research pool. The doctor-directed advertisements describing "instant cash" and "clinical research fame" become seductive. The typical, experienced, independent investigative site generated more than $1.1 million US dollars in annual net grant revenue in 1999.[1]

Today, the pharmaceutical industries are trying to reach peak sales faster and to extend product life cycle. The strategy of the companies is to rely on the investigators to increase the number of trials and provide future marketing input and selling initiatives. Success is not just about participating in an industry-sponsored trial: it is also about recruiting a large number of study patients. As competition has intensified, sponsors are vying for the top performing doctors by offering incentive monetary bonuses and gifts. Despite these incentives, most investigative sites believe that patient recruitment is much more difficult today than it was several years ago. On an average, only one patient for every 20 patients solicited, will complete a clinical trial.[1] This results in more pressure on the clinical investigator to perform.

Patients have become more knowledgeable about their disease and new therapies. This knowledge is obtained from direct to consumer advertisements of marketed product, Internet web sites, and lay press

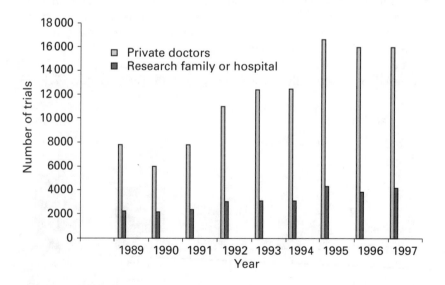

Figure 7.2   Number of new drug trials by location, 1989–97. (Source: *NY Times*)

describing new investigational trials. Patients are more motivated, more independent, and less trusting of a single medical opinion. These changes have resulted in patients who are increasingly receptive to clinical trials. In 1999 alone, 3.8 million study subjects participated (defined as screened and/or enrolled) in industry-sponsored clinical trials. Confidence among trial participants familiar with clinical research remains high, despite increasing numbers of complaints received by the FDA (Figure 7.3). Of the 13 clinical investigator complaints received by the FDA from sponsors in the fiscal year 1999, seven cases were related to potential data falsification.

In contrast, new patients and the general public have developed adverse views through the exposure to articles related to the misconduct of a few highly visible investigators and US Congressional Oversight hearings. Among the more recent examples of adverse clinical findings include the fraud perpetuated by Doctors Fiddes, Diamond and Borrison and the death of Jessie Gelsinger enrolled in a gene transfer trial at the University of Pennsylvania (see p. 109).

Each new case of scientific misconduct and fraud that makes its way into the public consciousness erodes away public trust in clinical research. Nevertheless the number of cases of scientific misconduct is small (average 3.4% of the total FDA audited cases, 1994–99) compared with the total number of academic and industry-sponsored research studies. When it does occur, it affects public confidence in the clinical trial process and raises questions about the effectiveness of trial monitoring and its follow up by sponsors. This is particularly valid with fraud because the clinical results have a direct impact on the treatment of patients. Media attention and US Congressional Oversight hearings devoted to fraud ultimately affect the careers of clinicians and their institutions as well as the overall management of research.

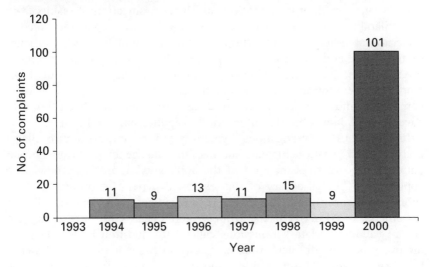

Figure 7.3   Complaints received by the FDA, 1993–2000.

107

What is research misconduct?

Research misconduct is fabrication or falsification in proposing, designing, performing, recording, or reviewing research, or in reporting research results. Research misconduct does not include honest error or honest differences of opinion.

In a report by the US Office of Research Integrity of 1000 investigations received between 1993 and 1997, falsification was the most frequent type of misconduct and accounted for 43% of the investigations.[2] In combination with fabrication[3] and/or plagiarism, falsification represents the most frequent type of alleged misconduct. Half of the biomedical researchers accused of scientific fraud in the US and subjected to formal investigations were guilty of misconduct.

Who commits fraud and their motivation?

Anyone who has access to or is responsible for collecting, transcribing, reporting, or monitoring data and is motivated to cheat may commit fraud. The motivations to commit fraud are as varied as human personalities.

Since the 1960s, more than 300 allegations have been reported to federal officials, including 40 clinical investigations audited by the FDA that have been classified as false information. Unfortunately, there is limited public awareness of fraudulent scientific/medical research (unless the information appears as newspaper headlines) and hence there is a limited outcry by the general public.

In the mid-1960s Industrial Bio Test (IBT) Laboratories "dry labed" many toxicology experiments, which led to the establishment of Good Laboratory Practices (GLP) regulations by the EPA and FDA.

In 1989, a series of investigations involving falsification of results from bioavailability studies of generic versions of innovator drug products led to the criminal indictment, conviction, and sentencing of several key officials at the FDA and generic pharmaceutical firms. As a result of those investigations, and investigations conducted by the FDA, four FDA employees were found to have accepted illegal gratuities from generic drug companies, and to date, 11 generic drug companies have been found to have falsified data submitted in premarket applications to the FDA.

In the FDA's investigations, which began as inquiries into illegal gratuities and questionable data submissions, the agency discovered broad patterns and practices of fraud in the applicants' abbreviated new drug applications. The discovery of this extensive pattern of fraudulent data submissions prompted the FDA to promulgate the Fraud, Untrue Statements of Material Facts, Bribery, and Illegal Gratuities policy[1] to ensure validity of data submissions called into question by the agency's discovery of wrongful acts, such as fraud, untrue statements of material fact, bribery, and illegal gratuities[2] and to withdraw approval of, or refuse to approve, applications containing fraudulent data.

Fraud in scientific research is not new, as articles elsewhere in this book show (See Chapters 4 and 5). At least five cases have involved court hearings. Barry Garfinkel, MD, a child psychiatrist at the University of Minnesota, was sentenced in 1994 to six months of home detention and ordered to pay $214 000 in fines and restitution, as well as 400 hours of community service for fraudulent studies in treating children and adolescents with obsessive–compulsive disorder.

John S Najarian, MD and Chairman of the Department of Surgery of the University of Minnesota, and Richard Condie, Research Director of the University, received a 55-count indictment in April 1995 for the illegal commercial sale and distribution of the investigational product, antilymphocyte globulin (ALG) and failure to report all deaths and serious adverse experiences to the FDA.

Bruce I Diamond PhD, a pharmacologist, assumed clinical research responsibilities and tasks for which he was unqualified and untrained. He received five years in jail; 10 years' probation; and was ordered to pay $1.2 million in restitution to the University System of Georgia.

Richard L Borison, MD, PhD, was sentenced to 15 years in jail; and 15 years' probation for the failure to personally conduct/supervise the investigation, failure to inform employees assisting in conduct of the studies of their obligations, and failure to maintain adequate and accurate records. He was fined $125 0000 and $4.25 million in restitution to the University System of Georgia.

Robert Fiddes, MD, President of the Southern California Research Institute, was sentenced in 1998 to 15 months in prison and ordered to pay $800 000 in restitution for the fabrication and falsification of over 200 studies sponsored by 47 drug companies.

US Government oversight in clinical research

For over half a century, the FDA and the National Institutes of Health (NIH) have been committed to protecting individuals from possible abuse or harm in clinical trials and to ensuring that prospective and enrolled subjects understand the potential risks and benefits in clinical research. The main mechanism of clinical research oversight is inspection. This commitment to protect subjects was the result of concerns, arising from the abuse of subjects, during the World War II trials at Nuremberg, the promotional distribution of thalidomide resulting in numerous children born with birth defects, the administration of cancer cells to chronically ill and senile patients at a hospital in New York, and others. In 1966, Henry Beecher brought prominent attention to human research abuses in medical schools and hospitals, citing 22 cases involving highly questionable ethics (and Maurice Pappworth did the same in the UK). The response of the US Government to Beecher's stories, led to amendments of the US Food, Drug and Cosmetic Act that required subjects to consent to participating in investigational research. In the 1970s, the National Commission for the Protection of

Human Subjects of Biomedical and Behavioral Research enhanced patient protection with recommendations for IRBs, ethical oversight committees that are responsible for ensuring that subjects who give consent to participate in clinical research fully understand the nature of the research and willingly consent to participate. The FDA revised its regulations in 1981 to require written informed consent in all studies of products that the FDA regulates.

In 1972, the Office for Protection from Research Risks (OPRR) was created as part of the NIH to ensure the safety and welfare of subjects who participate in Health and Human Services (HHS) sponsored research. Institutions engaged in human subject research must provide written assurance of compliance to the Regulations for Protection of Human Subjects (45 CFR Part 46). In 1999, the Advisory Committee to the Director of NIH recommended that the role of OPRR be expanded and that the office be elevated from NIH to HHS. In June 2000, the Office for Human Research Protections (OHRP) was established in the Office of the HHS Secretary to raise its stature and effectiveness.

The Food and Drug Administration (FDA)

The FDA must be assured that the rights and welfare of human subjects are adequately protected through compliance with applicable trial regulations. The results of studies on investigational new drugs will determine whether a drug will be approved by the FDA. Unlawful conduct, such as bribery and false statements pertaining to principal investigators, affects the integrity of the drug approval process.

Since 1977, clinical investigators, sponsors (that is, pharmaceutical companies), and Institutional Review Boards have been subject to inspection by the FDA Bioresearch Monitoring Program. All FDA product areas – drugs, biologics, medical devices, radiological products, foods, and veterinary drugs – are involved in the Bioresearch Monitoring Program. While program procedures differ slightly depending upon product type, all inspections have as their objective ensuring the quality and integrity of data and information submitted to the FDA as well as the protection of human research subjects. The objectives of these FDA audit procedures are to:

1   protect the rights and welfare of research subjects;
2   assure adherence to the regulations; and
3   determine the integrity of scientific testing and the reliability of the data in support of pending product approval by the FDA.

In 1999, the FDA financial disclosure regulations (21 CFR Part 54) were promulgated and became part of the expanded FDA inspectional procedures. The purpose of these regulations is to ensure that financial interests and arrangements of clinical investigators (that could affect the reliability of data) are identified and disclosed by the sponsor of the product. This information is obtained from the investigator before an investigator is allowed to participate. The penalty for not certifying and/or disclosing the financial information might result in the FDA refusing to file the market application (NDA).

Since the Investigational New Drug Regulations went into effect in 1963, the FDA has conducted over 6000 clinical investigator and 2000 institutional review board audits. Currently, the FDA is conducting over 400 inspections in the US (Figure 7.4) and 70 inspections outside of the country per year (Figure 7.5). To date, clinical data from 42 different countries have

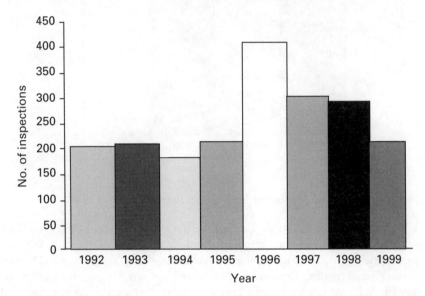

Figure 7.4   FDA inspections of US investigators, 1992–99.

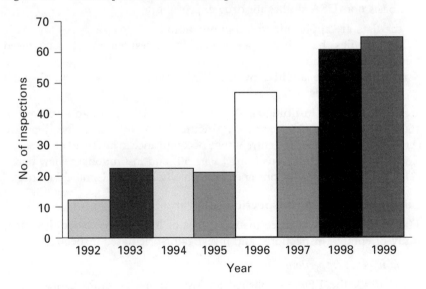

Figure 7.5   FDA inspections of non-US investigators, 1992–99.

111

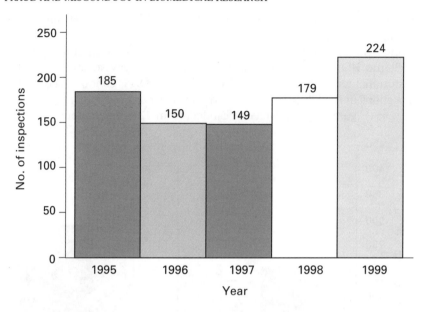

Figure 7.6   FDA inspections of Institutional Review Boards, 1995–99.

been inspected by the FDA. During the period of 1980–99, 380 non-USA inspections have been assigned in the following global regions: Western hemisphere (104), Europe–Japan–Australia–New Zealand (203), and former Eastern Bloc Countries (17). Non-USA studies may be audited by the FDA, if two USA adequate and well-controlled studies do not exist and international studies provide basis for drug approval. The FDA accepts as a sole basis non-USA studies for drug approval if:

1 the data are applicable to US population;
2 the studies have been performed by investigators of recognised competence; and
3 the studies are audited by the FDA or may be evaluated through appropriate means.

About 250–300 Institutional Review Boards (IRB) from an inventory of 1600 IRBs are inspected annually (Figure 7.6). The IRB inspections are performed to determine the current state of compliance to informed consent (21 Code of Federal Regulations [CFR] Part 50) and institutional review board (21 CFR Part 56) regulations and applicable ICH Good Clinical Practices.

Clinical investigator inspection programs

The FDA carries out three distinct types of inspections: bioequivalence, study-orientated inspections, and investigator-orientated inspections.

Bioequivalence inspections

From 1993, the FDA established an inspectional program to inspect *in vivo* bioequivalence studies (clinical and analytical components) supporting approval of marketing applications for generic drugs. The target of inspections are facilities new to FDA regulated research, high-volume facilities, facilities performing novel/non-conventional study procedures, and facilities with problems reported to the FDA.

Study-orientated inspections

FDA field offices conduct study-orientated inspections on the basis of assignments developed by headquarters staff. Assignments are based almost exclusively on studies that are important to product evaluation, such as new drug applications and product licence applications pending before the Agency. These assignments are based almost exclusively on studies that are important to product evaluation, new drug applications, and product licence applications pending before the FDA. Assignments may include pivotal clinical studies, studies where there have been an unusually high number of safety concerns or compliance issues raised by the sponsor, investigator, and/or the patient. Most FDA assignments are conducted on clinical investigators, whereas assignments on sponsors are relatively few. The FDA inspectional procedures and activities are described in the following FDA Compliance Programs: clinical investigators (CP 7348.811), sponsors (CP 7348.810), and institutional review boards (CP 7348.808).

The investigation consists of two basic parts. First, determining the facts surrounding the conduct of the study: who did what; the degree of delegation of authority; where specific aspects of the study were performed; how and where data were recorded; how test article accountability was maintained; how the monitor communicated with the clinical investigator; and how the monitor evaluated the study's progress.

Second, the study data are audited. The FDA investigator compares the data submitted to the Agency and/or the sponsor with all available records that might support the data. These records may come from the physician's office, hospital, nursing home, laboratories, and other sources. The FDA may also examine patient records that predate the study to determine whether the medical condition being studied was, in fact, properly diagnosed and whether a possibly interfering medication had been given before the study began. In addition, there may be a review of records covering a reasonable period after completion of the study to determine if there was proper follow up, and if all signs and symptoms reasonably attributable to the product's use had been reported.

Investigator-orientated inspections

An investigator-orientated inspection may be initiated because an investigator conducted a pivotal study that merits in-depth examination because of its singular importance in product approval or its effect on medical practice. An inspection may also be initiated because representatives of the sponsor have reported to the FDA that they are having difficulty getting case reports from the investigator, or that they have some other concern with the investigator's work. In addition, the FDA may initiate an

113

inspection, if a subject in a study complains about protocol or subject rights violations. Investigator-orientated inspections may also be initiated because clinical investigators have participated in a large number of studies or have done work outside their specialty areas. Other reasons include safety or effectiveness findings that are inconsistent with those of other investigators studying the same test article; too many subjects claimed with a specific disease given the locale of the investigation; or laboratory results outside the range of expected biological variation. The FDA may institute an investigator-orientated inspection for the following suspicious conditions: attempts to delay inspection; attempts to limit access to documents; investigator did it all himself; consent signature similarities; sudden tragedies (the "Titanic Phenomena"); notations out of chronological order and squeezed in between lines; and no original charts only photocopies of charts, ECGs, lab results.

Once the Agency has determined that an investigator-orientated inspection should be conducted, the procedures are essentially the same as in the study-orientated inspection except that the data audit goes into greater depth, covers more case reports, and may cover more than one study. If the investigator has repeatedly or deliberately violated FDA regulations or has submitted false information to the sponsor in a required report, the FDA will initiate actions that may ultimately determine that the clinical investigator is not to receive investigational products in the future.

After the site inspection, FDA headquarters usually issues a letter to the clinical investigator. The letter is usually one of four types:

- A notice that no significant deviations from the regulations were observed. This letter does not require any response from the clinical investigator ("classification NAI").
- An informational letter that identifies deviations from regulations and good investigational practice. This letter may, or may not, require a response from the clinical investigator. If a response is requested, the letter will describe what is necessary and give a contact person for questions ("classification VAI").
- A "warning letter" identifying serious deviations from regulations requiring prompt correction by the clinical investigator ("classification OAI"). In these cases, the FDA may inform both the study sponsor and the reviewing IRB of the deficiencies. The recipient of a warning letter is required to respond to the FDA within 15 working days. The Agency may also inform the sponsor if the clinical investigator's procedural deficiencies indicate ineffective monitoring by the sponsor.

In addition to issuing these letters, the FDA may take other courses of action, that is regulatory and/or administrative sanctions, including;

- A "Notice Inspection, Disqualification, Proceeding, and Opportunity to Explain (NIDPOE) Letter" issued when the FDA believes that it has evidence that an investigator has repeatedly or deliberately failed to comply or has submitted false information to the FDA or sponsor as described in 21 CFR 312.70. The NIDPOE letter informs the recipient clinical

Box 7.1 Basis for disqualification

- Repeated or deliberate submission of false data to the sponsor and the FDA (21 CFR 312.70)
- Failure to obtain IRB approval and comply with IRB regulation (21 CFR 56)
- Failure to obtain informed consent (21 CFR 50)
- Failure to sign investigator's statement form FDA 1572 (21 CFR 312.60)
- Failure to follow protocol (21 CFR 312.60)
- Failure to administer drug or under principal investigator supervision (21 CFR 312.61)
- Inadequate record keeping requirements (21 CFR 312.62)
  - drug dispensing
  - adequate case histories
  - record retention (2 years past FDA approval of NDA; 2 years post withdrawal of IND)
- Refuse to allow inspection of records by FDA (21 CFR 312.68)

investigator that the FDA is initiating an administrative proceeding to determine whether the investigator should be disqualified from receiving investigational products. The NIDPOE letter procedure was initiated in 1998.

Disqualification

The FDA may disqualify an investigator from receiving investigational drugs, biologics, or devices, if the FDA determines that the investigator has repeatedly or deliberately failed to comply with regulatory requirements for studies or has submitted false information to the study's sponsor. Investigators may also agree to certain restrictions on their conduct in future studies. Box 7.1 summarises the basis of disqualification and applicable FDA regulations.

Inspectional results

Food and Drug Administration

During the period from June 1977 to 31 December 1999, the number of study-orientated inspections and investigator orientated inspections represented 97% and 3%, respectively. The predominant clinical investigator deficiency categories for both USA and non-USA sites conducted during the fiscal years 1997–99 are described in Figure 7.7.

The FDA requires strict adherence by investigators to the protocol and documentation of data to show that the patients have met the protocol inclusion criteria and to permit evaluation of treatment response as well as a review of untoward adverse events. In the most serious cases, the failure to comply with the described protocol as approved by the institutional review

115

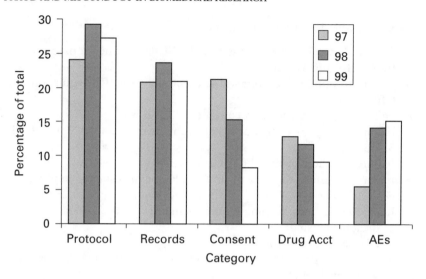

Figure 7.7   Clinical investigator deficiency categories, 1997–99.

board and submitted to the FDA may lead to rejection of data by the FDA and other regulatory agencies. In cases where the patient has been injured as a result of protocol violations, criminal prosecution can be initiated against the sponsor and/or investigator. Box 7.2 gives examples of protocol violations.

When deficiencies are identified by the FDA, a regulatory letter is sent to the investigator and the sponsor is advised that significant deviations from regulations were identified that require prompt voluntary correction. The identification of regulatory deficiencies or protocol violations does not necessarily constitute scientific misconduct or fraud. In the most serious regulatory deficiencies, the FDA may use one or more of the following regulatory administrative actions:

- Issuing a warning letter, which requires an investigator and/or sponsor response within 15 working days

Box 7.2 Protocol violations

- *Patient inclusion/exclusion criteria* – subjects listed as screened and non-qualifying
- *Concomitant medications* – the use of concomitant medications not approved in the protocol
- *Adverse reactions* – failure of the sponsor/investigator to report these observations on the contract report and transmit this information to the IRB and, when applicable, to the FDA
- *Data entry problems* – required data not entered on or missing on the contract report form; laboratory data incomplete or abnormal lab results not commented as required by the protocol

- Informing the sponsor that the study is not acceptable in a support of claims of efficacy in an application for research or marketing permit
- Sponsor inspection including termination of the IND application
- Initiation of the disqualification procedures or entry into a consent agreement with the clinical investigator
- Initiation of stock recovery by the sponsor
- Seizure of test articles if not exempted by regulation
- Injunction
- Prosecution.

The number of warning letters, NIDPOE letters and FDA action leading to investigator disqualification is illustrated in Table 7.1.

Disqualification, restriction, and prosecution

From 1964 to 1999, 99 investigators were disqualified (via hearing process or consent agreement) and became ineligible to use investigational products; 26 investigators were restricted for a limited time to receive test article through adequate assurance to the FDA; and 20 investigators were prosecuted or convicted (through consent agreement).

In 1998, the FDA began issuing a new type of regulatory letter – the NIDPOE letter, where the investigator had repeatedly or deliberately failed to comply or had submitted false information to the FDA. A total of 11 NIDPOE letters have been issued in fiscal years 1998–2000.

The FDA has identified several cases in which there was submission of false information (deficiency code 17). From June 1977 to 30 September 2000, there was a total of 40 domestic and two foreign investigators who submitted false clinical information (Figure 7.8).

Examination of recent cases of clinical research fraud in the US[3]

Dr Robert Fiddes, President of Southern California Research Institute, falsified multiple clinical studies during 1992–96. Dr Fiddes ignored protocol inclusion criteria and either enrolled patients into the trial by falsifying medical history and consequently endangering patients or

Table 7.1 FDA regulatory actions: clinical investigators.

Years	Warning letters		Disqualifications	Consent agreements	NIDPOE[a]
	Drugs & biologics	Medical devices			
1993–96	22	–	2	7	n/a
1997	3	10	0	1	n/a
1998	2	6	0	4	5
1999	10	4	2	5	2[b]
2000	13	10	0	0	5

[a]Notice of Initiation of Disqualification Proceedings and Opportunity to Explain.
[b]One resolved in favour of CI.

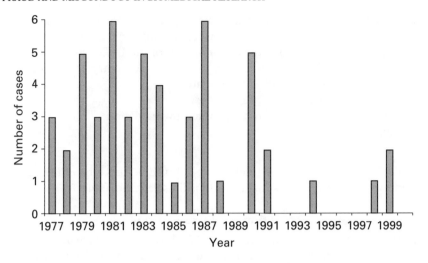

Figure 7.8   Submissions of false information audit, 1977–99.

enrolled fictitious patients by using employees of the research institute. In an ear infection study, the study protocol required subjects to have a certain bacterial infection. Study coordinators were directed to purchase the bacteria from a commercial supplier and shipped them to testing labs, stating that the specimens had come from patients. In a contraceptive drug study, Dr Fiddes substituted PAP smears from unidentified subjects for those from study subjects; blood from staff members was used to create lab work for three fictitious subjects; and subjects who dropped out were reported as completing the study. In a hypertension drug study, subjects were enrolled without required washout period, false ECGs created, and staff members instead of subjects wore Holter monitors. The Fiddes' scheme of fraud was well conceived. The company monitors and FDA personnel never noticed any problems with Fiddes' bogus paperwork, which they reviewed during routine audits. If it had not been for a disgruntled former employee, Dr Fiddes would have still been in business.

The authenticity of patients is highly suspect when investigators use bogus identities and use names from obituary columns (Dr S), or other investigators recycle subjects three to six times; or there are unopened cartons of the investigational drug identified with patient codes, and the CRF is completed after subjects died. In another case, Dr Lv signed the following affidavit based on FDA observations: "I, Dr Lv submitted false data on the majority of the patients in the following areas: 1. In at least 22 patients, identical sections of ECG tracings were submitted on different examination dates. 2. Radiological reports on at least 10 of 31 records submitted did not correspond with the initial examination date and/or not signed by the radiologist. 3. Diaries were in part filled in by myself (Dr Lv). 4. At least 23 of 31 endoscopy exams reported in the case report forms were not performed."

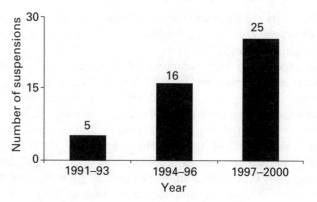

Figure 7.9   OPRR suspensions, 1991–2000. (Source: CenterWatch)

National Institutes of Health

About 1000 allegations of scientific misconduct were received by the NIH Office of Research Integrity (1993–97). Only 150 cases contained sufficient information to warrant further investigation. These cases resulted in 76 findings of scientific misconduct and 74 findings of no misconduct. The US Public Health Service (USPHS) imposed 170 administrative actions on the 76 respondents; 54 respondents (71%) were debarred from receiving Federal (USA) funding for periods ranging from 18 months to 8 years. Other actions included prohibition from USPHS advisory service (91%); supervised research (26%); certification of data (13%); certification of sources (9%); and correction or retraction of articles (13%).[4]

Since 1991, an increased number of institutions have been suspended by the US Government for violations of regulations and protocols (Figure 7.9). The Office for the Protection of Research has identified the following major problem areas: failure of the IRB to conduct continuing review at least once per year; failure of the IRB to review and approve protocol changes prior to their implementation; inappropriate use of expedited IRB review; failure of the informed consent documents to include adequate description of reasonably foreseeable risks and an adequate description of any benefits that may reasonably be expected.

Detecting scientific misconduct and fraud

The current system is designed to catch data errors, not detect fraud. The oversight system includes the responsibilities of the sponsor and the Institutional Review Board.

Responsibilities of the sponsor

Sponsors and their delegated representatives (that is, contract research organisations, site management organisations) are responsible for ensuring that clinical trials are conducted in accordance with FDA regulations. The FDA reports that monitoring is handled by sponsors (54%) and contract research organisations (31%).

A contract research that assumes any obligations of a sponsor must comply with the specific regulations (21 CFR 312.52[b]). The failure to comply with any obligation assumed will result in the same regulatory actions as will be taken with a sponsor. A sponsor who discovers that an investigator is not complying must promptly either secure compliance or discontinue shipments of the investigational new drug and end the investigator's participation in the investigation as well as notifying the FDA if an investigator's participation is under the [stated] conditions. The failure analysis of sponsor monitoring in recent notorious cases has identified the following problem areas:

- source documents completely absent;
- study subjects completely fabricated;
- study staff performing tasks for which they were unqualified; and
- other significant deviations from regulations.

To protect patient confidentiality, company representatives are instructed not to validate the existence of the patient through a review of clinic visit registrations and the accuracy of medical referral and history documents. As required in Section 505(i) of the Federal Food Drug and Cosmetic Act, companies require the establishment and maintenance of records and making reports by the sponsor as a condition for use of investigational drugs. Monitors need to insist on source data. Examples of source documents include medical history information; medical examination results; all lab results including x rays and ECG tracings; demographic data; concomitant medications; patient identification number; drug dispensing information; and informed consent. Too frequently, the sponsor will accept in lieu of source documents, shadow charts (summary medical information extracted from source data). Companies and their contracts need to have adequate time to review the integrity of data. Often monitoring time is truncated to allow more site visits in a given day, resulting in increased profits for the contract research monitoring organisations. Companies are eager to maintain a good relationship with the investigator and may replace monitors whenever the intensity of the data review becomes too rigorous. Unfortunately, there is no precise method for detecting if a doctor falsifies the underlying lab records or writes down inaccurate results for tests.

The sponsor is responsible for the selection of the clinical investigators based on the latters' training and qualifications, as evidenced by their *curriculum vitae*. The sponsor must certify that the data and information have been reviewed and are true and accurate. In addition, sponsors are required to certify financial interests and arrangements of the clinical investigator. Providing false statements represents a criminal offence (US Code Title 18, Section 1001).

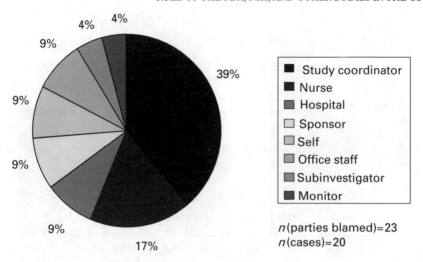

Figure 7.10   The blame game.

Excuses and the blame game

When scientific misconduct is identified, many individuals are blamed for the work and few, if none, take responsibility. In a review of responses to FDA inspectional observations, the type of people blamed for the shoddy work is illustrated in Figure 7.10.

Clinical investigators have created a number of excuses as to why records were not available for FDA inspection. Often the intentional missing record is a reason for suspicion. Experiences with clinical investigators have revealed the following explanations:

• "They were destroyed in a hurricane."
• "They were lost in a boating accident (burglary, robbery or vandalism)."
• "They were lost in the mail."
• "My father-in-law threw them out."
• "I do not see a problem with re-entering a patient five or six times (considering them as six different patients)."
• "I did not know that the medical charts and CRFs (data) must correspond."

Institutional Review Board oversight

All studies involving humans must be approved by an independent ethics board. The responsibilities of IRBs fall into two main categories: initial review and continuing review of research involving human subjects. The continuing review process seeks to ensure that the risk–benefit ratio of the research remains acceptable. The FDA recognises the important role of the IRB in implementing good clinical practice. However, in recent years, FDA inspection of IRBs has resulted in the identification of a number of

121

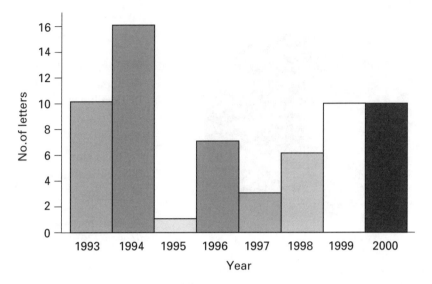

Figure 7.11   IRB warning letters, 1993–2000.

serious regulatory deficiencies. Among them include the lack of quorum for a committee meeting (25%); insufficiently detailed meeting minutes (21%); inadequate standard operating procedures (15%); and insufficient record keeping (10%). In the most serious cases, the FDA has issued warning letters to IRBs as illustrated in Figure 7.11. The US Office of the Inspector General report of 1998, described the IRB problems as; reviewing too much, too quickly with little experience; facing conflicts that compromise their independence; conducting minimal continuing review of approved research; providing little training for IRB members; and paying little attention to evaluating effectiveness.

In 1999–2000, the leading IRB problems evoking official action and issuance of a warning letter have been: failure to prepare and/or follow written procedures; failure to adequately document activities; failure to conduct adequate continuing review; failure to fulfil requirements for expedited review; and failure to fulfil the requirements of informed consent.

FDA activities

Investigator attitude and lack of cooperation as well as tip-offs from disgruntled employees are often early warning signs of fraud. The FDA rarely checks with patients and usually only when they have evidence of fraud. It becomes suspicious of the data when there are complaints from subjects, sponsors, or employees of the clinical investigator site; or there are too many subjects and efficacy and toxicity results that are "too good to be true".

If the FDA finds, on looking at fraudulent data in an application, that the data in the application are unreliable, the agency will exercise its authority, under applicable statutes and regulations, to refuse to approve the application (in the case of a pending application) or to proceed to withdraw approval (in the case of an approved application), regardless of whether the applicant attempts to replace the unreliable data with a new submission in the form of an amendment or supplement. Thus, if the applicant wishes to replace the false data with a new submission, the new submission should be in the form of a new application. The truthfulness and accuracy of the new application should be certified by the president, chief executive officer, or other official most responsible for the applicant's operations.

The FDA also may seek recall of marketed products and may request new testing of critical products. For drugs, for example, retesting may be requested for products that are difficult to manufacture or that have narrow therapeutic ranges. The FDA may pursue other actions, including seizure, injunction, civil penalties, and criminal prosecution, under the Food Drug and Cosmetic Act or other applicable laws, as necessary and appropriate.

Lessons learned

New efforts must be developed to improve human research safety and to reinforce clinical investigators' responsibility in the conduct of clinical research. Companies, institutional review boards, and clinical investigators must work in a collaborative manner to develop new policies on the prevention and detection of clinical research misconduct. Protection must be offered to persons identifying scientific misconduct. The whistleblower is an essential element in the effort to protect the integrity of clinical research, because researchers do not call attention to their own behaviour. Before making an allegation of research misconduct, a whistleblower should understand carefully to whom the allegation should be reported, what protections are provided for the whistleblower, and what part the whistleblower will play in future proceedings.

There are no specific rules for the detection of scientific misconduct and fraud. Nevertheless enhanced compliance with quality-orientated regulatory requirements for study conduct, reporting, and monitoring should allow its early detection. The quality-orientated regulatory requirements include clinical investigator and sponsor responsibilities. The former entails the conduct of the study performed in accordance with the protocol (21 CFR 312.60) and the maintenance of adequate and accurate case histories (21 CFR 312.62[b]). Protocol compliance requires the selection of a qualified clinical investigator and study coordinators as well as a commitment to continuous training and education. The sponsor requirements include proper monitoring of investigations (21 CFR 312.50), monitoring the progress of all clinical investigations being conducted under its IND (21 CFR 312.56[a]), and correcting and/or reporting serious non-compliance to the FDA (21 CFR 312.56[b]).

Failure to follow the protocol and to maintain adequate case histories continue to be the most frequently encountered FDA findings. Investigators must know that the data will be challenged both by regulators and the

123

sponsor. *Missing records may be a key indicator of potential fraud.* The integrity of clinical data requires original source documentation.

Sponsors need to provide adequate monitoring and independent quality assurance of their clinical trials including:

- adequate sampling of study sites;
- adequate sampling of time points throughout the trial;
- source data verification of data with no reliance on shadow records (that is, document what you did and did not do – if it is not documented, it did not happen);
- frequent monitoring and QA visits to resolve problems early;
- working together with contract research organisations to resolve differences.

Sponsors should:

- select exemplary investigators (qualified, experienced, interested, patient, committed, and able to deliver on time);
- review FDA inspectional information and select investigators who lack serious regulatory and protocol compliance issues and have corrected previous FDA observations;
- educate and train clinical investigators at preclinical investigation meetings as well as investigator responsibilities;
- select qualified, knowledgeable, and reliable contract research organisations (CROs) and monitors;
- review FDA inspectional material.

Identification of scientific misconduct requires the preparation of a complaint handling system by both sponsors and investigators to capture, document, and deal with complaints of misconduct in a timely manner. The procedures for complaint handling should be defined in a policy (that is, Standard Operating Procedure document) that relates to the receiving, reviewing, reporting, and processing of complaints. Confidentiality of the whistleblower should be described. All complaints should be *assumed* to be credible unless demonstrated to the contrary after thorough evaluation and supervisory review and approval. Follow-up activities are required for all complaints and should be categorised on the basis of the highest priority of reports related to gross abuse of subjects' rights that result or have the potential to result in death or injury. The system should be carefully monitored to ensure timely evaluation and final resolution. The FDA believes that complaints should be reported whenever there is a discovery of misconduct and not delayed when the clinical investigator has been dismissed. Clinical research team members are encouraged to recognise and report research misconduct to government agencies.

Recognising scientific misconduct and fraud requires education and training. In addition to understanding current trial regulations and responsibilities of investigators, ongoing training is needed to learn about problems with investigators and the sharing of knowledge of trial sites.

Accessibility to government information websites has aided in the knowledge of scientific misconduct. The Food and Drug Administration and the Office of Research integrity have posted on internet websites the names of investigators who have been disbarred/restricted and related public health service (PHS) administrative actions. Information can be accessed through the FDA Home Page: www.fda.gov/ora/compliance.ref/default.htm

Investigator, IRB, sponsor warning and NIDPOE letters are accessible on the FDA website as well.

Conclusions

Now is the time to move beyond misconduct as an academic subject and devote more attention to incorporating better clinical research practices to identify and prevent research fraud. These practices include a partnership of the clinical investigator, institutional review board, and the sponsor. Clinical investigators, corporate managers, and individuals alike would do well to re-examine their own practices for warning signs. The failure to adopt a vigorous approach will lead to new cases of research fraud and ultimately erode away public confidence in the research enterprise.

References

1   CenterWatch, November 2000.
2   Food and Drug Administration. Freedom of Information Office, FDA, Washington DC, USA.
3   Food and Drug Administration. *Guide to detecting fraud in bioresearch monitoring inspections, April 1993*, FDA.
4   Department of Health and Human Services, Office of Research Integrity. *Scientific misconduct investigations report (1993–1997)*, DHHS.

8: The Danish committees on scientific dishonesty

HANS HENRIK BRYDENSHOLT

Establishment

In the autumn of 1992, the Danish Medical Research Council established a Danish Committee on Scientific Dishonesty.[1,2] A High Court Judge was appointed as chairman on the recommendation of the President of the High Court, and seven members were appointed on suggestion from institutes of higher education concerned with medical research, the Joint Committee of Directors of government research institutes, the Association of Local Governments, as well as the Danish Medical Society. The members, who all had recognised health science expertise, were appointed for a 3-year period. When this first period expired, the work of the committee was evaluated favourably and the Ministry of Research took over the responsibility for the future financial support. The original committee continued its work until the end of 1998. At this time new legislation was passed and an organisation covering fraud in all scientific fields was formed.

The work of the original committee (1992–98)

The committee did not have the power to make decisions that were legally binding. It could only investigate cases and express its opinion. So the research community was not given the power of self-governance, as is the case, for instance, for lawyers and certified accountants. Nevertheless, the conclusions of the committee were taken extremely seriously by the persons and institutions involved, given that its members were recognised opinion leaders in the research community.

Formally the committee was not part of the public administration, and hence not subject to the Freedom of Information Act. As it was considered important that the details of the case would not appear in the press while the investigation was ongoing, the committee decided not to give public access to documents before the parties were told of the decision.

From the very start, the committee considered that it was important to conduct its business in such a way that the parties would not need to be represented by lawyers. If a party should wish to be represented by a professional organisation or a private lawyer, he or she should be free to do so, but it was considered to be unfortunate if it became regular practice to involve lawyers, so as to avoid any replication of the legalistic development seen in the USA.

The Committee dealt with all aspects of scientific dishonesty in medical science. Dishonesty includes all deliberate fraudulent work at any time during the application-research-publication process, as well as such extreme cases of negligence that the question of professional credibility becomes an issue. This corresponds to the legal concepts of intent and gross negligence.

Self-evidently such a definition was rather strict. In the years 1992–98, when the committee received 45 complaints and investigated 25 cases, dishonesty was found in only four cases. Nevertheless, the committee did not restrict itself to concluding whether dishonesty was found or not. It used another norm in that, when it thought that the behaviour had violated good scientific practice, it said so in its conclusion of the case. For example, the committee has stated that a researcher acted against good scientific practice when he publicly presented research results which at the time had not yet been published in the usual scientific way. In its view, prior to presentation to the public, a research paper should undergo peer review and discussion in the research community. An aggravating circumstance was when a researcher publicly discussed not his own but another researcher's unpublished work.

The question has been raised whether fundamental legal principles are jeopardised when, at one and the same time, the committee decides which acts should be regarded as contrary to good scientific practice and then uses its own defined norms as the basis for its decisions. A fundamental tenet has always been that legal rules cannot be used before they have been published so that the public can become aware of their existence. In response to this criticism, the committee emphasised that it did not itself decide the norms for good scientific practice. It has always referred to what the opinion leaders in the scientific community have generally regarded as unacceptable behaviour – what, to speak legally, could be described as customary law. When the decisive point is whether the norms were recognised beforehand by opinion leaders, it is evident how vital it is that the members of the committee are recognised as leading figures in the profession. Fortunately the members have had this status, and the activity of the committee and its decisions have generally been acclaimed by the research community and society at large.

Another question has been why the committee has gone beyond what its statutes defined as scientific dishonesty. For what reason was the norm regarding violating good scientific practice introduced? The reason was that typically any breach of good scientific practice will create tensions among researchers, and bad personal relationships in small research units can be extremely damaging for the institution's performance. Thus to maintain a standard of good scientific practice will not only protect the interest of individual researchers against unfair behaviour from competing fellow researchers, but also protect the institutions against behaviour that could give rise to an unproductive, hostile interrelationship among the employees. Once again it should be emphasised that the committee has not looked upon itself and its practice as normative, but as a body which crystallises and formulates norms already recognised by opinion leaders in the field.

Examples of scientific dishonesty in medicine

Three of the cases,[2] where the original Danish committee found scientific dishonesty, are summarised as follows:

Case 1 – The author of a paper published in a Nordic journal discovered an abstract on MEDLINE with an identical title and data. The abstracted paper originated from a foreign journal. Plagiarism was established, and the paper was retracted. Later on, more than 20 papers were found to have been plagiarised by the same person, who was dismissed from his professorship.

Case 2 – A senior registrar published research results from his work at a clinical department without the permission and knowledge of his superiors, and he included them as authors without their knowledge. The registrar was dismissed.

Case 3 – An American information company offered a Nordic expert the authorship of a completed review paper recommending a certain drug. The company was wilfully dishonest since it attempted to give the impression that the review was impartial, and because it broke the rules for authorship (ghost authorship). The name of the company was disclosed in the committee's yearly report.

Terms of reference for the new committee system established in 1999

In 1998 a frame law was passed that empowered the Danish Minister of Research to create committees on scientific dishonesty, covering all research fields. Pursuant to that in December 1998 the Minister published a regulation "Concerning the Danish Committees on Scientific Dishonesty" with the following provisions:

The Board of the Danish Research Councils establishes three committees on scientific dishonesty within Danish research: a committee covering natural science, agricultural and veterinary science and technical science, a committee for health and medical science, and a committee for social science and the humanities. The committees will share a chairman, whose task among other things is to ensure uniformity in the statements made by the committees irrespective of the scientific issue in question ...

It is the responsibility of the Danish Committees on Scientific Dishonesty to handle cases concerning scientific dishonesty when the Committees receive complaints thereof. A plaintiff may ask the Committees to consider his/her case in order to clear his/her name of circulating rumours and allegations. The case must be of importance to Danish research. If it is unlikely that the Committees will find for the plaintiff, the complaint will be dismissed, before actually being considered by the Committees.

Scientific dishonesty includes actions or omissions in research, such as falsification or distortion of the scientific message or grossly misleading information or actions regarding a person's efforts within the research and include, e.g.:

1 Construction of data
2 Selective and hidden rejection of undesirable results
3 Substitution with fictive data
4 Deliberately misleading application of statistical methods
5 Deliberately distorted interpretation of results and distortion of conclusions
6 Plagiarism of other people's results or publications
7 Deliberately distorted representation of other people's results
8 Inappropriate credit as author
9 Incorrect information on applications.

In order to characterize behavior as scientific dishonesty, it must be documented that the accused has acted with intent or gross negligence regarding the activities under consideration.

A complaint of scientific dishonesty must be submitted within a reasonable time after the plaintiff has obtained the necessary basis for lodging the complaint. Only in special cases, will the committees consider cases concerning activities dating back five years or more.

If a committee concludes that scientific dishonesty has taken place in a specific case, it may:

1 Inform the accused person's employer
2 Recommend that the scientific work in question be withdrawn
3 Report to the public authority, supervising the area
4 Report to the police in case of penal code violation
5 Make a statement about a possible choice of sanction, upon special request by an appointing authority.

The committees will publish annual reports on their activities. The reports will describe all considered cases of scientific dishonesty, without indicating the names of individuals or institutions involved. (It is practice to publish the reports in Danish and English.).

The chairman must be a High Court Judge. The appointed members and their alternates must be recognized researchers who together cover the scientific areas of the Danish Research Councils as broadly as possible. The chairman and the members are appointed in their personal capacity.

The chairman is appointed by the Minister of Research and Information Technology. The members and the alternates are appointed by the Board of the Danish Research Councils upon the recommendation of the Danish Research Councils.

The individual committee may decide that the handling of a case requires the assistance of one or several external experts.

The committees will attempt to reach unanimous decisions. If this is not possible, decisions are reached by majority vote. A dissenting member may request to have his/her dissent noted in the conclusive statement.

The committees' handling of cases falls under the Danish Administrative Law.

Experiences under the new committee system

Apart from the chairman, each of the committees has only four appointed members. This is a weakness, given that authority of the committees relies entirely on the recognition of its members as opinion leaders in their respective research fields. Especially in medicine, research covers such a huge and diversified area that it is necessary to draw on more experience than the appointed four members represent themselves. So the committee dealing with medical science has decided to invite also the alternate members to participate in its meetings. That their participation – under the rules of the committee – is without voting power is of no significance. It is the participation in the discussion of personalities with a wide experience in research that is so valuable.

Another weakness is that the rules of the committees have no provision for preventive work. Even so, all the committees have recognised this as part of their responsibilities, and to fulfil this task, have questioned the universities and institutes of higher education about the kind of knowledge junior researchers get in this field. Later on, the committees will prepare information material to be used in the education of junior researchers.

It would have also been helpful, if the rules had contained a provision regarding exemption from the Freedom of Information Act. However, all the committees have decided not to give the public (the media) access to documents during the investigation. In a case decided upon in 2000 a journalist complained to the Danish Ombudsman about this practice, and the complaint is still under consideration.

Finally, even if most complaints still relate to medical research in medicine, in 1999 and 2000 there were complaints referred to the committee covering natural science and to that dealing with social science and the humanities.

All the committees have decided to decide on not only whether a behaviour is dishonest or not, but also whether the accused has shown behaviour contrary to good scientific practice. It is premature to say whether the norms in the various research areas will be the same. This is one of the reasons why it is found necessary to have one or two meetings in a year where all the members and alternates from the three committees are called for a common discussion.

References

1 Brydensholt HH. The legal basis for the Danish Committee on Scientific Dishonesty *Science and Engineering Ethics* 2000;**6**:1–14.
2 Nylenna M, Andersen D, Dahlquist G *et al.* Handling of scientific dishonesty in the Nordic countries. *Lancet* 1999;**354**:57–61.

9: Scientific fraud and misconduct in Finland

VEIKKO LAUNIS

There is one national ethics committee in Finland dealing with the prevention, handling, and investigation of scientific dishonesty, The National Research Ethics Council of Finland. The Council was founded in 1991 and is subordinate to the Ministry of Education. The Council consists of a chairman, a vice-chairman, a secretary general, and eight members who represent researchers, jurisprudence, and ethics. The Council is appointed for three years by the Ministry of Education. In the Decree on the National Research Ethics Council of Finland (1347/1991), the following tasks are assigned to the Council:

- to make proposals and to issue statements to governmental authorities on legislative and other matters concerning research ethics;
- to contribute, in its expert capacity, to resolving issues of research ethics;
- to take initiative in promoting research ethics and discussion on research ethics;
- to follow international development in the field and take an active part in international cooperation;
- to raise awareness of research ethics in the society at large.

As regards the handling of alleged scientific dishonesty, the Finnish research community has adopted an approach different from that existing in other Nordic countries.[1] The Finnish system is *decentralised*. The Council does not itself investigate cases of alleged or suspected scientific dishonesty, but, in 1998, produced *Guidelines for the Prevention, Handling and Investigation of Misconduct and Fraud in Scientific Research*. According to these guidelines, universities and research institutes are responsible for preventing scientific misconduct and for investigating suspected or alleged cases of scientific dishonesty. The investigative procedure includes an *initial inquiry* (conducted by the rector of the university or the director of the research institute) followed, if necessary, by a *full investigation* by a specially appointed committee. The committee reports to the rector of the university

131

or the director of the research institute who will make a decision on implementation of any sanctions and on measures necessary to rectify the consequences of fraud or misconduct. Three principles are considered to be essential in ensuring the fair treatment of all parties: *impartiality*, the *hearing of all parties* and the *promptness of the process*.

The Research Ethics Council is informed of all inquiries and investigations, and receives the final report on each case. If either the researcher involved or the informant is dissatisfied with the proceedings or with the result of the investigation, they can request an opinion from the Council. The role of the Council is advisory, and it does not issue legally binding decisions.

Misconduct and fraud in science: defining the concepts

Misconduct in science

The reliability and dignity of scientific research are based on the expectation that researchers comply with good scientific practice. While the full meaning of "good scientific practice" is open to discussion, the concept is agreed to include at least the following: "adherence to procedures accepted by the scientific community, general conscientiousness and accuracy in the performance of research and presentation of results, appropriate acknowledgement of the work and achievements of others, honest presentation of the researcher's own results and respect for the principles of openness and controlled procedures of science."[2] Violations of good scientific practice (misconduct in science) include "underestimation of the contribution of other scientists in one's own publications, insufficient reference to results achieved earlier, sloppy and therefore potentially misleading reporting of methods or results, inadequate documentation and insufficient preservation of data, covert duplicate publication and any conscious attempt to mislead the general public with regard to the work of the researcher in question."[2]

Fraud in science

By "fraud in scientific research" the Research Ethics Council refers to the presentation to the scientific community of fabricated, falsified, or misappropriated observations or results, for example in a presentation held in a scientific meeting, a manuscript written for the publication, or a research grant application. *Fabrication* includes reporting invented observations not based on the methods presented in the research report or entirely imaginary results based on no actual observations. *Falsification* of scientific observations means "intentional alteration of data or the presentation of observations in a manner which alters the end result." Falsification of results means "altering or selecting the results of the research in a scientifically unjustifiable manner." Falsification thus also involves the exclusion from a report of results essential to the findings of the research.

Table 8.1 Specification of cases according to accusation.

Alleged dishonesty	1998			1999			2000		
	A	B	C	A	B	C	A	B	C
Plagiarism				5	4	1	1	0	1
Adoption of the original research idea, a research plan, or research observations	3	3	0	4	3	0			
Fabrication or falsification of scientific observations	1	1	0	1	1	0	2	1	0
Falsification of application documents or scientific merits				2	2	0			
Misconduct in science	2	1	1	1	0	0	7	1	0
Other				6	2	0			
Total number of cases	6	5	1	19	12	1	10	2	1

A = cases handled in the universities and research institutes.
B = cases handled by the Research Ethics Council.
C = dishonesty proved.

Also included in fraud is "the adoption of the original research idea, a research plan or research observations of another researcher" (*misappropriation*); or "the presentation, either as a whole or in part, of a research plan, a manuscript, article or other text created by another researcher as if it originated from the researcher in question" (*plagiarism*).[2]

The prevalence of scientific dishonesty in Finland

In 1998, the Finnish universities and research institutes handled six new cases of suspicion or accusation of scientific dishonesty. In 1999, the number of new cases was 19, and in 2000, 10. Between 1994 and 1997, 12 new cases were reported. So far, 47 cases have been reported. In eight cases, scientific dishonesty was revealed. Whilst the number of accusations and suspicions has increased dramatically during the 1990s, the proved cases of scientific fraud or misconduct are very few (approximately one per year). Specification of cases according to accusation is given in Table 8.1.

Though the proportion of the number of cases handled by the Council to the number of cases handled by universities and research institutes has decreased during the past few years, it is too early to say how effectively the decentralised system works.

References

1 Nylenna M, Andersen D, Dahlquist G, Sarvas M, Aakvaag A. Handling of scientific dishonesty in the Nordic countries. *Lancet* 1999;**354**:57–61.
2 The National Research Ethics Council of Finland. *Guidelines for the prevention, handling and investigation of misconduct and fraud in scientific research.* Helsinki. Ministry of Education, 1998.

10: Experiences of fraud and misconduct in healthcare research in Norway

MAGNE NYLENNA

Since 1994 there has been a National Committee for handling scientific dishonesty in healthcare research in Norway. A wide definition of dishonesty has been applied including "all serious deviations from accepted ethical research in proposing, performing and reporting research". Eleven alleged cases have been investigated so far, disputed authorship being the single most frequent reason for complaint. Dishonesty has been revealed in only two instances, but the Committee has undertaken several preventive efforts and has developed a coherent system for handling future cases of suspected misconduct.

Background

The National Committee for the Evaluation of Dishonesty in Health Research in Norway (The National Committee) was established in September 1994 by the Medicine and Health Division of The Research Council of Norway. This was preceded by a report from a working group appointed by the Research Council in December 1992.[1] This report drew extensively on a Danish account[2] and recommended the founding of a permanent national body. The idea of a national committee on scientific dishonesty met some resistance in Norway in the early 1990s. Among the most critical was the Norwegian Researchers' Association, expressing concern for the legal protection of researchers accused of misconduct. A number of individuals, including some prominent scientists, also questioned the need for such a committee. "Most researchers will realise that it is unethical and silly to publish results that are not founded on honest and precise research. Very soon experiments will be checked or repeated in other laboratories. If one finds that they are wrong and based upon dishonesty, the career of the person in question will be restrained by itself without anonymous hints and without any witch-hunt."[3]

134

On the other hand, investigations indicated that dishonest conditions did exist in Norwegian health research. In a questionnaire distributed to 119 project leaders, nearly 40% responded that fraud in health care was a problem. More than every fourth respondent said that he or she was aware of concrete instances of misconduct, and 18% claimed that they themselves had been exposed to misconduct.[4] In another questionnaire, 22% out of 219 researchers reported that they were aware of serious violations of research-related ethical rules; 3% knew of instances involving the fabrication or falsification of results in their immediate research environment, while 10% believed that plagiarism or the theft of results had occurred, and 9% had themselves contributed to one or more of the conditions defined as scientific misconduct.[5]

The National Committee was given two main goals: to prevent scientific dishonesty, and to ensure that reported alleged incidents of scientific dishonesty in the health sciences are investigated. The statutes included a wide concept of dishonesty defined as "all serious deviations from accepted ethical research in proposing, performing and reporting research." This has later been specified as "serious, intentional or grossly negligent violations of accepted ethical research in proposing, performing and reporting research." According to its statutes, the National Committee investigates cases upon the agreement and on behalf of the employer of the accused person. It reports the findings to the relevant institution and the involved parties, and leaves any sanctions to the employer. Anonymous complaints are, in principle, rejected and there is no formal appeal mechanism. The National Committee includes representatives from several healthcare professions: physicians, a dentist, a pharmacist, a psychologist, as well as a judge.

Experiences

Promoting preventive measures has been given high priority by the National Committee. General information on ethics in research and publication has been disseminated to relevant institutions, and the Committee has cooperated with university faculties on the teaching and content of doctoral courses, seminars, and lectures. The topics of dishonesty, ethics, and good publication practice are now included in the compulsory coursework for doctorates in Norway.

The Committee has arranged open conferences on *Scholarly publication – the author's responsibility and merits* and on *Good and bad practices in researcher training*. Ethical problems in the relationship between supervisor and research fellow have been given specific attention. Conflicts in this field often revolve around authorship and the ownership of data.

National guidelines for the implementation of research projects related to medicine and health have been produced and distributed to researchers and research institutions. The objective of these guidelines is to prevent disagreements among project participants and prevent doubts from being raised about the implementation of a project.

135

From September 1994 to September 2000 a total of 11 cases of alleged dishonesty were accepted for investigation (see Box 10.1 at the end of this chapter). One case was withdrawn and another case has been referred to the National Committee in Denmark because of conflicts of interest among the members of the Norwegian Committee. Investigations have been undertaken by *ad hoc* committees reporting to the National Committee, which decides on a conclusion. To increase the educational and preventive values of the decisions, a practice has developed not only to base the conclusions on a dishonesty/non-dishonesty judgment, but also to describe explicitly in what way a non-dishonest practice is found to deviate from good scientific practice.

Eight cases have been closed. In two cases the accused was completely cleared, in three cases minor deviations from accepted ethical research were found, and in two cases the committee concluded that scientific dishonesty had taken place.

In addition to the formal complaints the Committee as well as its individual members have been consulted in several instances by researchers and institutions on issues regarding research and publication ethics.

The national committees on scientific dishonesty in the Nordic countries cooperate closely, and, even though there are slight differences in working procedures and the definition of dishonesty, the experiences are fairly similar.[6]

Discussion

Roughly one new investigated case of alleged dishonesty per year in a country with 4.5 million inhabitants, four medical schools, and 18 000 physicians seems low and this gives cause for reflection.[7] The most probable explanation for the low figure may be summarised by four hypotheses:

- The most obvious explanation is that there simply are no more cases than the few reported in Norway. This does not, however, fit with national surveys.[4,5] Moreover, anecdotal accounts and confidential inquiries indicate that there is at least a suspicion of dishonesty on many occasions.
- In spite of its six years' history, the existence of the National Committee is not sufficiently well known. Experience from other countries shows that press coverage in the wake of major disclosures helps to make such committees widely known. As there have been no major cases in Norway in recent years, the media coverage of the activities of the committee has been modest.
- The committee, and its methods, do not enjoy sufficient confidence. The committee does not define what constitutes "accepted research ethics" but builds on the understanding the committee members have of accepted research ethics in Norway. Thus the members must have a knowledge of the research community as well as its confidence. Even though the scepticism towards the committee has diminished over the years, it still exists.

- Potential complainants hesitate to report cases because of fear of jeopardising their career. It is well known that whistleblowers may end up worse off than the person who engaged in the misconduct.[8] The National Committee in Norway does not consider anonymous inquiries and a complainant must be prepared to be identified and be held publicly accountable for the complaint.

The presumption of misconduct is the core of any case, but the mere existence of misconduct or the suspicion of dishonesty does not in itself initiate an investigation. There must be a complaint and most likely the complainant will be involved in or related to the case in one way or another. Often there is a particular situation that triggers the complaint. Such "situations" may include competition, disagreement, jealousy, or other interpersonal relations. Without a "situation" suspected or even obvious, cases of dishonesty might not be reported and investigated.

A small number of investigated cases and even fewer cases of verified dishonesty may be seen as an argument against the existence of a national system for dealing with scientific dishonesty. A score of cases gives, however, the minimum of experience that is needed to handle possible future events. The cooperation between the Nordic countries exchanging information and meeting on a regular basis adds to this experience. Last but not least, the number of cases investigated and disclosure of misconduct is not the only and perhaps not even the most important measure of success. The preventive work at a national level and the existence of the Committee in itself might have a prophylactic effect.

The resistance against a national body for dealing with scientific dishonesty has gradually declined in Norway during the last decade, even though some scepticism still exists. Nevertheless, from the Norwegian experience a coherent system for handling of misconduct based on a broad definition combined with preventive efforts is feasible and effective.

Box 10.1 Cases investigated by The National Committee for the Evaluation of Dishonesty in Health Research in Norway

1. Two new co-authors had been included on a scientific paper without consulting the other authors according to the complainant. Even though the committee found that one of the authors did not fully qualify for authorship, it did not characterise this as a serious violation of ethical research practice.
2. Claims of unreliable measuring methods, publication of mis-interpreted data, erroneous statistical analyses, and unqualified co-authorship were made in a research project. Scientific dishonesty could not be established but the committee underlined the importance of good routines for laboratory practice and keeping logs, and for clarifying authorship.

3. The complaint concerned a researcher's contribution to a government report. The main points of the discussion were whether the work that had been done was research or the reporting of research. The complaint was withdrawn and accordingly no final decision was taken by the committee.

4. A researcher had presented results to the general public in a press interview without prior scientific presentation according to the complainant. The committee found that the results had been presented scientifically prior to the interview and that the incident did not represent scientific dishonesty.

5. A researcher was accused of plagiarism in a textbook. The committee found that the case showed a deviation from accepted practice in terms of research ethics. The breaches were found to be blameworthy but, viewed as a whole, not sufficiently serious to be characterised as scientific dishonesty.

6. The case involved a conflict between a former research fellow and the research group represented by the research fellow's supervisor. The research fellow wanted to patent a technical invention that was part of the research group's work. The supervisor rejected this idea, but the research fellow continued to try to get a patent, partly in secret from the rest of the research group. The committee found the research fellow's actions to be dishonest.

7. This was a claim made by two researchers against a third colleague, who allegedly neglected to include several patients in a study in which they were registered and to report serious side effects observed in several of the patients in the same study. This case is currently under consideration.

8. This case refers to a complaint about the presentation of a preliminary report without accessible scientific documentation and of suppression of other findings. The committee concluded that there had been no withholding or distorting of data in the preliminary report, even if the analyses had been insufficiently performed. The committee criticised the researcher for not publishing the article in full until many years later, but did not find him dishonest.

9. The first author of a paper published in an international journal had included several Norwegian co-authors who had not taken part in the study and without their knowledge or consent. The committee concluded that the publication represented a serious offence against accepted norms and procedures of scientific publication and was considered scientific dishonesty.

10. A junior researcher made a complaint against a senior researcher, who did not accept the publication of an article based on data collected at the hospital where the senior was in charge. According to the senior researcher, the data were not collected in a proper way

and there was no protocol for the project. This case was referred to the Danish Committee, which concluded that the senior researcher had the right to stop the publication and that the actions were not unethical.

11. A junior researcher accused a professor of claiming authorship in a scientific paper without being involved in the research. According to the complaint the junior researcher was not allowed to publish the study without including a senior who did not qualify for authorship. The case is still under investigation.

References

1 Norges forskningsråd. Uredelighet i helsefaglig forskning (*in Norwegian*). [The Research Council of Norway. Dishonesty in health research.] Oslo: The Research Council of Norway, 1993.
2 Andersen D, Attrup L, Axelsen N, Riis P. *Scientific dishonesty and good scientific practice.* Copenhagen: The Danish Medical Research Council, 1992.
3 Iversen OH. Om fristelse til uredelighet i helsefaglig forskning. Kuren må ikke bli verre enn sykdommen (*in Norwegian*). [On the temptation to engage in misconduct in health research. The cure must not be worse than the disease.] *Tidsskr Nor Laegeforen* 1994;**114**:230–1.
4 Hals A, Jacobsen G. Uredelighet i medisinsk forskning (*in Norwegian*). [Dishonesty in medical research.] *Tidsskr Nor Laegeforen* 1993;**113**:3149–52.
5 Bekkelund SI, Hegstad A-C, Førde OH. Uredelighet i medisinsk og helsefaglig forskning i Norge (*in Norwegian*). [Dishonesty in medical and health research in Norway.] *Tidsskr Nor Laegeforen* 1995;**115**:3148–51.
6 Nylenna M, Andersen D, Dahlquist G, Sarvas M, Aakvaag A. Handling of scientific dishonesty in the Nordic Countries. *Lancet* 1999;**354**:57–61.
7 Nylenna M. Why are so few cases reported to the National Committee? In: *Dishonesty in health research. Report on the National Committee's work from 1994 to 1997.* Oslo: The Research Council of Norway, 1998.
8 Kohn A. *False prophets. Fraud and error in science and medicine.* Oxford: Basil Blackwell, 1988.

11: Dealing with misconduct in science: German efforts*

STEFANIE STEGEMANN-BOEHL

In 1997 the German scientific community was stirred by strong suspicions that 47 papers by two high-flying cancer researchers, Friedhelm Herrmann and Marion Brach, included fabricated data.[1] So far, misconduct in science had been considered a sign of decadence of the New World. But all of a sudden, the topic aroused the interest of prestigious German research organisations as well as of journalists, deans, rectors, presidents, and even public prosecutors. Several local commissions and a joint commission investigated the case. Marion Brach confessed to journalists that a mix of sex, violence, and intrigue – which according to her statement must have been typical for the relationship between Herrmann and herself – was the cause of what had happened. She lost her job in Lübeck. Herrmann was suspended from his job in Ulm and then quitted it, before any further disciplinary actions were taken.

History

Misconduct

The Herrmann and Brach scandal – sometimes called the "fall of German science"[1] – certainly marks a turning point in the history of misconduct in Germany. "Gemütlichkeit" in German research suddenly became a thing of the past, but, the history of misconduct in science in Germany actually starts in the 1920s in Berlin, if not much earlier, in the 19th century.

In the second half of the 19th century, the German Zoologist Ernst Haeckel published his notorious graph showing embryos of different vertebrate animals that – at a certain stage of their development – look alike, but the graph turned out to be manipulated. It did not show different embryos but only one embryo, shaped by Haeckel from case to case according to his needs.[1]

*The following account reflects the author's personal view.

More than 40 years later, Albert Einstein is supposed to have manipulated research data by not disclosing relevant experimental data that did not harmonise with his theory. Later on, the undisclosed data turned out to be the relevant ones.

The next documented case of fabrication and falsification of data is that of the Berlin physicist Ernst Rupp, who published spectacular experiments in the 1920s and 1930s on the interference of electron beams – experiments that were, without exception, fictitious.[2,3]

In the 1930s, the Berlin biologist Franz Moewus manipulated data in his doctoral thesis about seaweed. Later on, as a professor in Heidelberg, he investigated the genes of a special sea plant and presented to the scientific community spectacular results that were forged. His fraudulent behaviour was detected in the 1950s in Australia, where he went after the war.

Hasko Paradies had earned international recognition for his publication on the crystallisation of transfer RNA, and had been appointed to the chair of plant physiology and cell biology at the Free University of Berlin in 1974. In 1982, it became known that his publications were based on falsified data. The university set up a committee of enquiry. In 1983, Paradies reached an agreement with his employer that he would himself ask to be dismissed from permanent civil servant status, whereupon the university undertook not to investigate the case further.[2,3]

Another case, which caused a great international stir, was that of the British biochemist Robert Gullis, who, in 1974 and 1975, as research fellow at the Max-Planck Institute for Biochemistry in Martinsried near Munich, fabricated research results on neurotransmitters. His group published several articles based on the fictitious results.[4]

From the 1980s a couple of "nameless" cases and rumours have been reported, such as the case of a doctoral student in Braunschweig who invented data that he needed for his dissertation in chemistry and doctored his lab book. The doctoral degree was taken away when the manipulations were detected.

The "Lohmann" case dates back to 1993. The Giessen biophysicist Lohmann had been accused of having published results on skin cancer research that his colleagues thought did not stand up to closer scientific scrutiny. A co-worker complained about discrepancies between the measuring results obtained at the institute and those published by Lohmann. Unfortunately, Lohmann had lost his primary data. An *ad hoc* committee set up by Giessen university investigated the case and obliged Lohmann to publish errata and to stop using specific data henceforth. Lohmann sued the university, and the administrative court as well as the appellate court, and the Federal Administrative Court held that the suit was founded, though for different reasons. Whereas the lower courts ruled that university committees are generally not allowed to apply sanctions to scientists, the Federal Administrative Court ruled that this is possible as a matter of principle; in this specific case, however, the committee had exceeded its limits. The final revision by the Federal Constitutional Court of 8 August 2000, did not change the ruling of the Federal Administrative Court.[5-9]

Another spectacular case even had political implications: in November 1993, much too high air–benzol values were found in southern Germany. To counter this, officials planned a couple of traffic restrictions, but in February 1995 the data were found to have been falsified. The person who had guided the benzol study is supposed to have increased the test results by 30% in order to place the results of his dissertation in a better light.[10]

In 1994, a working group of the chemical department at the University of Bonn claimed to have discovered that certain chemical reactions can be controlled by magnetic fields. The results were published in a professional journal and met with a favourable response within the scientific community. Suspicion arose, though, that Guido Zadel, a doctoral student might have forged them. He is under suspicion of having added the desired reaction products to the original solution, deceiving in this way also his co-workers who were to examine his results. The student was fired. His head-of-the-lab dissociated himself from the results in a letter to the journal. Bonn University decided to take the doctoral degree away from the student, who had been honoured for his work. Since 1997, the case has been pending at the administrative court of Cologne.[11]

Plagiarism

Plagiarism in science is not unknown in Germany either. As early as 1957, disciplinary proceedings were instituted against a professor who had included work written by a staff member in his own publications without informing the staff member or giving him authorship. The proceedings were eventually suspended because the professor was found by the court only to have been negligent.[12]

A court ruling in 1961 was based on a case in which an educationalist, in a book on national socialist education, had plagiarised the explanations on the educational theory of Ernst Kriek published 16 years earlier by a scholar in the same discipline.[13]

In the 1970s, a doctoral student of biology took her supervisor to court because he had disseminated the results of her – as yet unpublished – dissertation in a scientific treatise.[14]

Another example of plagiarism in science led to a court ruling in 1980.[15] The state examination thesis of a biology student had been chosen for publication in a scientific series because of its outstanding quality. A dispute ensued because a staff member of the chief editor intended to add a few scientific evaluations and, for this reason, wished to be named as co-author. The examination candidate did not approve of his request and demanded his work back, upon which the staff member of the editor published a paper which – with the exception of some additional evaluations – was almost identical in content and structural organisation, if not in the wording, to the examination candidate's thesis. No reference whatever was made to the student, who sued the editor's staff member for infringement of copyright. The suit was dismissed in the last instance by the Federal Court of Justice (Bundesgerichtshof).

In 1981, a historian was also refused copyright protection. He had gone to court because his work on border conflicts – supposed to have taken place according to the national socialists at the German Polish border immediately before the outbreak of World War II – had been included in a book without acknowledgement of source, almost literally and *mutatis mutandis*.[16] The plagiarist was none other than a public prosecutor, who was at the time involved in his official capacity in one of the incidents reviewed and was permitted by the historian to draw on the unpublished manuscripts for his investigations.

In 1993, the rector of Essen University, Horst Gentsch, had to resign, because parts of his inaugural speech were copied (without reference) from another person's essay, which had appeared two years earlier.

In 1986, a professor of mathematics had his teaching licence taken away for deceit after it had become known that his thesis was almost identical to a monograph originally published in Russian but meanwhile, unfortunately, translated into English. The professor sued against the revocation of his licence to teach, but was unsuccessful in two instances.[17,18]

The "Ströker" case,[19–21] which attracted attention in the press, had a different outcome. The Cologne professor of philosophy, Elisabeth Ströker, was accused by her colleague, Marion Soreth, of copying from other works in her doctoral thesis. Bonn University – where Ströker had obtained her doctorate – decided not to take away the doctoral degree. The argument was that, at the time Ströker did her doctorate, it was general practice to provide fewer references than today, in particular when reporting other authors' views. A complete list of references at the end of the dissertation – as was included also in Ströker's thesis – was therefore sufficient.

Finally, a couple of incidents of misuse of the peer-review system have also become known – or rather, half-known – in Germany.[1] Much public interest was aroused by the confession of Marion Brach, that Herrmann and herself had misused their position as peers by advising the rejection of a grant application (submitted in English), and then submitting more or less the same application (translated into German) as their own shortly afterwards to the same funding agency.

Epidemiology

After the Herrmann and Brach case had become notorious, more cases of suspected misconduct became publicly known than had previously. Some of them probably cannot be taken too seriously.

In 1997, Martin Schata, a specialist in allergic illnesses at the University of Witten-Herdecke and President of the German Allergy and Asthma Union, was under suspicion of having manipulated data in his studies about mites. Nevertheless, the accusations seemed insubstantial and presumably personally motivated.

Another probably personally motivated campaign was that of Bernhard Hiller against Jens Rasenack, a Freiburg professor of medicine. Hiller alleged – also via the internet – that the former head of his laboratory made use of manipulated data. Although an expert appointed by the University of Freiburg concluded that Hiller was mistaken, he stuck to his opinion.

However, some other cases are more serious. Roland Mertelsmann, a specialist in gene research at Freiburg University, came under suspicion of having participated in the fraudulent behaviour of Herrmann and Brach, as he is the co-author of 25 incriminated papers. An investigative commission of the university concluded that Mertelsmann had not actively forged data, but had neglected his supervisory duties.[22]

Soon after the Herrmann and Brach case became public, there was a rumour in the media about Thomas Lenarz, a specialist in ear, nose, and throat diseases in Hannover, having claimed scientific pioneer work for himself that a colleague had done before. Lenarz was admonished by the university.

Also, the case of Meinolf Goertzen from Düsseldorf has been publicly discussed since 1997. Goertzen is under suspicion of having published manipulated figures, which he denies. A legal procedure is pending.

Another case happened at the Max-Planck Institute for Psychiatry between 1991 and 1996. A young researcher had continuously forged and invented scientific data in his publications and, on one occasion, stolen results from a colleague. He was relieved when he was detected, spoke about personal difficulties, withdrew his thesis, and resigned from a future academic career.

In 1998, data manipulations in a project of a working group of the Max-Planck Institute for Plant Breeding in Cologne became public. According to the results of a Max-Planck investigation, a technician was responsible for these, but the laboratory head was also held responsible, because he never monitored the results – not even when suspicion arose. Thus, both resigned.

In 1999, Peter Seeburg, working then at the Max-Planck Institute for Medical Research in Heidelberg, was held culpable of misconduct committed in 1978. In the latter period he had worked at the University of California at San Francisco, where he was busy cloning genes. Later, he changed to a firm that did gene research, and, to continue this research, he stole the material from his former laboratory. Finally, his firm applied for a patent. The Max-Planck Commission held that stealing items required for research cannot be tolerated because this disturbs the atmosphere of confidence between researchers. Secondly, Seeburg did not tell the truth about the production of the clone in a paper based on the research that led to the patent.[23,24]

The latest case is that of the Erlangen philosopher Maximilian Forschner, who copied, in his book about the "fortune of mankind", large passages from his Oxford colleague James Urmson's book *Aristotle's ethics* without quoting it. His behaviour was officially criticised as misconduct by his university.[25,26]

Aetiology

The causes of misconduct in science have often been debated. As in other countries, in Germany the publish or perish principle, honorary authorship, impact factor fetishism, and the situation of graduate students faced with the choice of condoning, or actively participating in, their superior's misconduct, or leaving the group to face an uncertain future, have all been incriminated as promoting misconduct.[27]

The conditions under which researchers work in Germany should help to reduce the problem. Here, the academic research community and the social security of the researchers are far less dependent on grants than, for example, in the USA.[29] With only a few exceptions, universities and scientific research institutions are either state maintained or receive basic government funding. Being government employees or civil servants, researchers can, to a certain extent, conduct research from the basic funding available to their institution, but the share of university research paid for from external funds is increasing, above all in the natural sciences. Furthermore, although applicants in Germany do not have to make a living by raising funds, they do have to provide for some staff members, a fact which – apart from the wish to carry out a certain project – can be no less an incentive to lower the "conscience threshold" too much when making an application. Hence self-evidently the German system is not immune against misconduct, although the temptation to engage in it might be weaker than in certain other countries.

Investigation and management

A couple of years ago, Germany had no special rules regarding misconduct in science.[28–30] There was a complete lack of institutional safeguards for promoting good scientific practice and for dealing with infringements. This did not mean that norms and rules, developed for other types of illegal activities, such as the provisions against fraudulent behaviour, could not be applied to misconduct in science – provided that those immediately affected did not settle the problem in private, as was done in most cases. Rules developed for other types of illegal activities could – and can still – be applied, but this did not ensure that misconduct could always be handled efficiently.

The prosecution of misconduct as fraud, for example, will usually fail except in particularly blatant cases. One reason for this is that the prosecution of minor cases will fail for lack of evidence. It would be very difficult, for example, to prove that a researcher wanted to deceive a funding agency with at least conditional intent, to give rise to an error, and to cause a theft stemming from that error, but unless all this is proved, he cannot be punished for fraud. In a civil procedure, a researcher cannot be sure of being able to prove that he has been wronged, and risks losing the case and having to pay any associated costs. As for plagiarism, the German system has to deal with the problem that papers are protected only against unlawful literal copying. The scientific content – in particular, the research result, and thus that which is most important to the researcher – does not enjoy copyright protection. If a researcher is stimulated to carry out research work of his own by a peer's work that he is reviewing, the researcher who has submitted the manuscript or grant application has no means of protecting himself.

In addition, if one excludes disciplinary action towards civil servants, there is no other opportunity to react to misconduct in a less than major way. A minor manipulation of data, for example, may not be sufficient to give a funding agency the right to end a funding relationship retrospectively. A minor plagiarism may not be sufficient grounds for dismissing a researcher. Thus, employers and funding agencies have no chance of reacting adequately to minor cases of misconduct.

This is the gap intended to be filled by new regulations proposed by two very important German research institutions and funding agencies. Since the Herrmann and Brach case has upset the German scientific community, there is a consensus that the topic "misconduct in science" cannot be shrugged off with a "*mundus vult decipi*". On the contrary, pressure upon research and funding institutions has grown considerably to deal with such matters properly.

Nevertheless, even before this case, procedures for handling allegations had been drawn up by the most prestigious German funding agency for academic research, the German Research Foundation (Deutsche Forschungsgemeinschaft – DFG[31]), – in 1992 – and they were then revised in 1999.[32] Only months before this, the Max-Planck Society (Max-Planck Gesellschaft – MPG)[33] also presented a set of regulations.[34] Subsequently the latter have served as a pattern for the revised procedures of the German Research Foundation as well as for the model procedure[35] of the German Rectors' Conference (Hochschulrektorenkonferenz – HRK),[36] which its member institutions gradually translate for their own purposes. In addition, the Helmholtz Centers of Research[37,38] and some professional associations[39–41] are currently addressing the problem. Finally, the German Federal Ministry for Education and Research (Bundesministerium für Bildung und Forschung (BMBF)) plans to oblige its beneficiaries to accept the standards of good scientific practice.

Most of the new regulations recommend the appointment of one or more experienced members of the academic staff as ombudspersons. These latter are supposed to react to accusations and to pursue on their own initiative any clue of possible academic misconduct. An ombudsperson should also advise whistleblowers confidentially and examine the changes in terms of their credibility. Beyond this, in July 1999 the German Research Foundation appointed an "Ombudsman for Science" with a nationwide responsibility to advise and assist scientists and scholars in questions of good scientific practice and its impairment through scientific dishonesty.[42]

Most of the new regulations enable special investigative committees to check, in two-stage proceedings consisting of an informal inquiry and a formal investigation, whether or not allegations of misconduct can be upheld or, in the case of professional associations, be used to exclude members on the basis of misconduct.

Unlike for example, Denmark, every institution has its own committee. Thus, the system of dealing with misconduct in science in Germany is strictly local, being neither centralised as in Denmark, nor having a controlling institution such as the Office of Research Integrity in the United States.

The investigative committees have the mandate to establish the facts of the case and to form a reasoned opinion on whether or not misconduct has occurred. If a committee concludes that misconduct is not proved, it closes the case. If it concludes that misconduct has occurred, it informs the leadership of the institution (for example, the rector of the university; the President of the Max-Planck Society), and recommends further action that will then have to be taken by the institution (for example, warning, notice of termination of employment, withdrawal of a degree). An appeal stage is deliberately avoided, because it would extend the time needed to reach resolution. In any case, a scientist to whom sanctions have been applied can always appeal through the courts. Therefore, cases of serious misconduct will invariably end there.

Most of the new regulations deem academic misconduct to have occurred if, in a scientifically significant context, false statements are made knowingly or as the result of gross carelessness; if the intellectual property of another is violated; or if their research activities are otherwise disadvantaged. Examples of misconduct – as given in the regulations – are:

- *False statements* (for example, invention of data; falsification of data, such as by selecting and withholding unfavourable results, without disclosing this or by manipulating a diagram or illustration; the supply of incorrect information in an application or in a request for funds, including false information regarding the publication body or publications in press).
- *Violation of intellectual property* (with respect to a copyright work of another person or the significant scientific findings, hypotheses, theories or research methods of others; the unauthorised exploitation involving usurpation of authorship – plagiarism; the misappropriation, particularly in an expert opinion, of research methods and ideas – theft of ideas; the usurping of scientific authorship or co-authorship, or the unjustified acceptance thereof; the falsification of the contents or the unauthorised publishing and making accessible to third persons of work insight, hypothesis, theory or research method not yet published; the assertion of the (co-)authorship of another person without his or her consent).
- *Impairment of the research work of others* by the sabotage of research work (including damaging, destroying or manipulating research arrangements, equipment, documents, hardware, software, chemicals, or other items required by another person for carrying out an experiment).
- *Joint accountability* (joint accountability may, *inter alia*, be the result of active participation in the misconduct of others, of having knowledge of

147

falsification committed by others, of co-authorship of publications affected by falsification, and of gross neglect of supervisory duties. The special circumstances of each are decisive).

Compared with other countries, the circumstances under which research and funding institutions are allowed to appoint a misconduct committee appear to be restrictive:

- According to the ruling of the Federal Administrative Court from 11 December 1996 in the "Lohmann" case summarised above,[43] institutions of higher education may call upon the services of a committee to examine the circumstances of a case of suspected misconduct only if there is definite evidence that a scientist may be abusing his academic freedom, or jeopardising or violating the rights of others. Mere scruples about the academic work of a scientist are not sufficient. In the actual case, the university had to deal with mere scruples and therefore did not have the right to set up a committee. Thus primary data that corresponded to the irreproducible results of Professor Lohmann's were lost. Therefore, definite evidence that he used wrong data was missing. The scruples of his colleagues would have had to be the subject of controversial scientific debate, not of the work of a university committee.
- A committee may act only on the matters in question and only if and to the extent that serious charges are brought against a scientist. A serious charge may be that the scientist acted irresponsibly in breach of the fundamental principles of scholarship; that he has abused the principles of academic freedom; or that there is reason to question the academic nature of his work, not only in special regards or according to the definition of a special school, but on a systematic basis.
- The committee is authorised to make an appropriate statement and to criticise the work of the researcher to the extent that he is found undoubtedly to have overstepped the limits of the freedom of science. If, however, the academic seriously endeavours to respect the principles of academic work, and has likewise not violated the rights of others, the committee must not pass judgment on the work in question.
- The supervisor responsible for disciplinary action is to be informed of any disciplinary offence and should then take further action. If the rights of another have been violated, the committee has to take the necessary action to protect those concerned.
- Confidentiality has to be respected. The standards should be those of formal disciplinary proceedings.

The reason for these restrictions is article 5 paragraph 3 of the German Constitution, that stipulates: "Art and science, research and teaching shall be free." According to the interpretations of this article, which have been developed by the Federal Supreme Courts for Administrative, and particularly for Constitutional, affairs over the decades, scientists are given herewith an individual right to honest error and a right to pursue scientific ideas that differ from the mainstream. Any official action (which includes university action or the action of a public funding agency) that might imply censorship of scientific ideas is forbidden. Article 5 paragraph 3 of the Constitution also has to be respected if a scientist is suspected of misconduct – a behaviour, that is itself not protected by Constitutional law – as such a suspicion might well be unjustified. Therefore, special misconduct investigations are allowed only between the boundaries mentioned above.[44]

It may be a characteristic of the German management of misconduct that German institutions care much about isolating and repairing damage to the research community incurred by scientific fraud.[45] To separate truth from lies in the Herrmann and Brach affair, the German Research Foundation and the Mildred Scheel Foundation charged an investigation group with tracing the history of the fabricated data in 550 papers and 80 book chapters. In June 2000, the group concluded that at least 94 scientific publications by Herrmann and 54 publications by Brach contained fraudulent data, and that another 121 Herrmann publications were suspected of containing fictitious data.[46] Similarly, the Max-Planck Society required its Institute for Plant Breeding in Cologne to repeat all the experiments reported in papers that had relied on assays that were manipulated.[45]

To safeguard good scientific practice, reactive measures are indispensable but not sufficient. Preventive measures must also be introduced. To begin with, an attempt might be made to make researchers more aware of the problem of misconduct through workshops and ethics instruction. Thus, in its model procedure, the German Rectors' Conference encourages the faculties to cover the subject of academic misconduct in a suitable manner within the curriculum to raise the awareness of students and young academics to such issues.

In addition, the *Proposals for safeguarding good scientific practice*[47] of the German Research Foundation are an important help for German research institutions and scientific societies that recognise their institutional responsibility and seek to tackle misconduct in science. The Herrmann and Brach case had led the Executive Board of the German Research Foundation to appoint an international commission with the mandate of exploring the causes of dishonesty in the science system; to discuss preventive measures; to examine the existing mechanisms of professional self-regulation; and to make recommendations on how to safeguard the latter. As the result of its deliberations, the commission has put forward the *Proposals for safeguarding good scientific practice*.

Furthermore, the idea of reducing the pressure to publish by limiting to a low maximum number the publications required for filling the vacancies ("Harvard Scheme") has had some positive response in Germany[48] and I hope that this attitude will spread.

Although the German Research Foundation and also the Max-Planck Society were lucky to have misconduct procedures when the Herrmann and Brach case (respectively, the Seeburg and the technician case) became public, there still seems to be a reluctance in Germany towards accepting misconduct guidelines. Even nowadays, applause is certain for anybody who conjures up the terrors of the notorious bureaucratic overkill;[22] the confidence of researchers in the "self-healing powers" of science is still very strong, but the experience of the last years shows that the legendary self-healing powers definitely have to be initiated and guided by special principles.[22]

Given the multiple sets of misconduct procedures and statements on good scientific practice in Germany over the last few years, there is some hope that misconduct will be successfully tackled. In particular, one hopes that the "spirit" of these guidelines will be accepted throughout the scientific community.

References

1 Finetti M, Himmelrath A. *Der Sündenfall – Betrug und Fälschung in der deutschen Wissenschaft.* Stuttgart: Raabe, 1999.

2 Fölsing A. *Der Mogelfaktor: Die Wissenschaftler und die Wahrheit.* Hamburg: Rasch und Röhring, 1984.

3 Eser A. Misrepresentation of data and other misconduct in science: German view and experience. In: Cheney D, ed. *Ethical issues in research.* Frederick, MD: University Publishing Group, Inc, 1993, p. 73–85.

4 Andersen D, Attrup L, Axelsen N, Riis P. *Scientific dishonesty and good scientific practice.* Copenhagen: Danish Medical Research Council, 1992, p. 27–8.

5 Verwaltungsgericht Giessen. Verdict III/V E 651/91, 23 February 1993.

6 Hessischer Verwaltungsgerichtshof. Verdict 6 UC 652/93, 23 February 1995.

7 Bundesverwaltungsgericht. Verdict 6 C 5.95, 11 December 1996. *Neue Juristische Wochenschrift* 1997, p. 1996.

8 Bundesverfassungsgericht. Verdict 1 BvR 653/97, 8 August 2000.

9 Stegemann-Boehl S. Stein der Weisen oder Steine statt Brot? Grundsatzentscheidung des Bundesverwaltungsgerichts zu Betrugsvorwürfen in der Wissenschaft. *Frankfurter Allgemeine Zeitung* 7 May 1997, N1.

10 Behr A. Benzol-Alarm mit falschen Zahlen. *Frankfurter Allgemeine Zeitung* 10 February 1995: 11.

11 Flöhl R. Chemie in Magnetfeldern. *Frankfurter Allgemeine Zeitung* 13 July 1994: N1.

12 Dienststrafhof für die Länder Niedersachsen und Schleswig-Holstein. *Deutsche Verwaltungsblätter* 1957:461.

13 Landgericht München I. *Archiv für Urheber-, Film-, Funk- und Theaterrecht* 1961;35:223.

14 Landgericht Köln. *Archiv für Urheber-, Film-, Funk- und Theaterrecht* 1977;78:270.

15 Bundesgerichtshof. Gewerblicher Rechtsschutz und Urheberrecht 1981:352.

16 Oberlandesgericht Frankfurt/Main. Verdict 15 U 198/80, 27 August 1981.

17 Verwaltungsgericht Arnsberg. *Mitteilungen der Kultusministerkonferenz zum Hochschulrecht* 1989:170.

18 Oberverwaltungsgericht Nordrhein-Westfalen. *Nordrhein-Westfälische Verwaltungsblätter* 1992:212.

19 Soreth M. *Kritische Untersuchung von Elisabeth Strökers Dissertation über Zahl und Raum nebst einem Anhang zu ihrer Habilitationsschrift.* Köln: P und P, 1990.

20 Soreth M. *Dokumentation zur Kritik an Elisabeth Strökers Dissertation.* Köln: P und P, 1991.

21 Ströker E. *Im Namen des Wissenschaftsethos – Jahre der Vernichtung einer Hochschullehrerin in Deutschland 1990–1999.* Berlin: Berliner Debatte Wissenschaftsverlag, 2000.

22 Eser A. Die Sicherung von "Good Scientific Practice" und die Sanktionierung von Fehlverhalten mit Erläuterungen zur Freiburger "Selbstkontrolle in der Wissenschaft". In: Lippert H-D, Eisenmenger W, eds. *Forschung am Menschen. Der Schutz des Menschen – die Freiheit des Forschers.* Heidelberg, New York: Springer, 1999.

23 Stegemann-Boehl S. Skandalträchtige Klone – Die Ethik des Heidelberger Molekularbiologen Peter Seeburg. *Frankfurter Allgemeine Zeitung* 26 May 1999; N1.

24 Peter Seeburgs Verhalten offiziell missbilligt. *Frankfurter Allgemeine Zeitung* 15 December 1999; N2.
25 Schulz M. Glücklicher Schwindel. *Der Spiegel* 30/2000. http://www.spiegel.de/spiegel/ 0,1518,87156,00.html.
26 *dpa-Dienst für Kulturpolitik* 39/2000, 25.9.2000, p. 21.
27 Schneider C. Safeguarding good scientific practice; new institutional approaches in Germany. *Sci Engineering Ethics* 2000;**6**:49–56.
28 Stegemann-Boehl S. *Fehlverhalten von Forschern – eine Untersuchung am Beispiel der biomedizinischen Forschung im Rechtsvergleich USA-Deutschland.* Stuttgart: Enke, 1994.
29 Stegemann-Boehl S. Fehlverhalten von Forschern und das deutsche Recht. *Wissenschaftsrecht* 1996;**29**:140–60.
30 Schmidt-Aßmann E. Fehlverhalten in der Forschung – Reaktionen des Rechts. *Neue Zeitschrift für Verwaltungsrecht* 1998;1225–42.
31 http://www.dfg.de
32 Verfahrensordnung der Deutschen Forschungsgemeinschaft zum Umgang mit wissenschaftlichen Fehlverhalten.
33 http://www.mpg.de
34 Max-Planck-Gesellschaft zur Förderung der Wissenschaften e.V., Verfahren beim Verdacht auf wissenschaftliches Fehlverhalten. Procedure in cases of suspected scientific misconduct. 1997. For full details see http://www.mpg.de/fehlver.htm (German); http://www.mpg.de/fehlengl.htm (English).
35 Zum Umgang mit wissenschaftlichem Fehlverhalten in den Hochschulen. Dealing with academic misconduct in institutions of higher education. Resolution of the 185th plenary session, 6 July 1998. For full details see the HRK homepage (publications – plenary statements – 185th plenary session).
36 http://www.hrk.de
37 http://www.helmholtz.de
38 Hermann von Helmholtz-Gemeinschaft Deutscher Forschungszentren. Sicherung guter wissenschaftlicher Praxis und Verfahren bei wissenschaftlichem Fehlverhalten. 10 September 1998 (Framework regulation; regulatory statutes have been enacted by some but not by all HGF-member institutions).
39 Gesellschaft Deutscher Chemiker (1994) requires scientific integrity of its members.
40 Deutsche Physikalische Gesellschaft (1998) establishes rules on publication and good scientific practice.
41 Fachgesellschaft der Ärzte in der pharmazeutischen Industrie: "golden memory". cf. Schwarz J. Fehlverhalten und Betrug bei klinischen Prüfungen. *Die pharmazeutische Industrie* 1996;**58**:1097–105.
42 http://www.dfg.de/aktuell/info_wiss...Archiv/info_wissenschaft_26_99.htm.
43 Cf Lippert BM. Dealing with academic misconduct in Germany. *Professional Ethics Report* 1999;**XII**(2):1,7,8.
44 The question of the power of ethical commissions in general is analysed by Gramm C. Ethikkommissionen: Sicherung oder Begrenzung der Wissenschaftsfreiheit? *Wissenschaftsrecht* 1999;**32**:209–25.
45 Science comes to terms with the lessons of fraud. *Nature* 1999;**398**:13–17.
46 Finetti M. Forscher fälschten fleißiger als bisher bekannt. *Berliner Zeitung* 20 June 2000.
47 Deutsche Forschungsgemeinschaft. *Vorschläge zur Sicherung guter wissenschaftlicher Praxis. Proposals for safeguarding good scientific practice.* Weinheim: Wiley-VCH, 1998. Also available under http://www.dfg.de/aktuell/download/selbstkontrolle.htm; http://www.dfg.de/ aktuell/download/self_regulation.htm
48 Albert-Ludwigs-Universität Freiburg. "Selbstkontrolle in der Wissenschaft", 16 December 1998, Part I, 5.(3). An interpretation of these guidelines is in reference 22.

12: Fraud and misconduct in medical research in France*

JEAN-MARC HUSSON, JEAN-PAUL DEMAREZ

"The physician supplied too many guinea pigs" This article of a daily newspaper is about a GP charged with fraud, forgery and use of forgery, at the request of Agence Française de Sécurité Sanitaire des Produits de Santé (Afssaps).
France-Soir, 15 December, 2001[1]

Introduction

Because medicinal products are the most highly controlled and sensitive of healthcare products, European and national health authorities have a very active role to play in combating fraud. Despite the harmonisation of drug development, registration, evaluation, and monitoring in Europe since the early 1960s, and the creation of the European Agency for the Evaluation of Medicinal Products (EMEA) in 1995, rules to control the specific problem of fraud in clinical research have not yet been commonly addressed and implemented. Neither the European Commission nor the national agencies have specific passages about fraud in medical research in their pharmaceutical regulations. The new European Parliament and Council Directive, published in May 2001, relating to the implementation of good clinical practice in the conduct of clinical trials,[2] addresses indirectly the question of fraud, but only by referring to the "credibility of data" through the ICH (International Conference on Harmonisation) GCP text.[3] There are no specific sections on properly managing fraud once it is suspected.

France, as one of the 15 member states of the European Union, has agreed to develop quality assurance systems as well as national inspection programmes, as called for notably by such directives. The EMEA inspection unit has only a co-ordinating role between member states; it is charged to establish European inspection rules and methods, but has no right or possibilities for any direct inspection, which remains at the national level only.

*This chapter is dedicated to Professor Eigill Hvidberg (DK), "Father of the European GCP" texts, who has recently died.

In France, the notion of fraud is codified only in the general legislative texts that cover all activities (for example, civil or criminal law). In principle, silence is the general and, in practice so far, the official and professional golden rule. Such absence of clear and specific legislation about fraud in biomedical research may explain the few official reports on fraud. Thus there are no official figures for the prevalence of fraud in clinical trials on drugs/medicinal products, which come under the responsibility of the "Agence Française de Sécurité Sanitaire des Produits de Santé" (Afssaps), even though a figure of 2% has been reported elsewhere.[4]

In spite of the creation of the European Union nearly 50 years ago, there are still profound cultural differences between member states, and this is shown by the diversity of their approaches to fraud. Clearly common rules must be adopted so that each country can communicate uncontaminated data to the others. It is not a question of interfering with issues specific to each country, but rather of allowing harmonisation of working rules so that results achieved by one country are acceptable to all.

Concepts

The nature of fraud, possibly defined in the French language as "*Un acte de mauvaise foi et de tromperie accomplie en vue de nuire au droit d'autrui*," is described elsewhere in this book. In the case of falsification of scientific or clinical data, this type of fraud tries to modify the benefit risk/ratio and the therapeutic value of a new specialty to be submitted for a Marketing Authorisation (AMM in France), by improving the data. It has consequences in terms of both public health and public finance (when this new agent is reimbursed by the social security system). The origin of the fraud can be within the pharmaceutical company itself. Consequently, a marketing authorisation granted by Afssaps on falsified data, could be judged as illegal and subsequently cancelled. Marketing authorisation can also be considered as invalid and withdrawn, if the fraud was achieved outside and without the knowledge of the company.

A sponsor organising a fraud is committing a forgery, and this is envisaged and penalised in article 441-6 of the new French *code pénal* (criminal code). Whatever its degree, importance, or systematisation, any fraud is considered a fraud – that is, deceiving "*a moral person by using fraudulent operations*" – penalised in article 313-1 of the new criminal code. In any legal action against the investigator or his/her partners, the pharmaceutical company is justified in asking for (financial) compensation, according to the importance of the damage done (delay in the marketing authorisation, or the necessity for a new study to be carried out).

When an informed consent form has been falsified the new code includes a specific infringement if a study subject is enrolled in a study without written consent or maintained in the study after withdrawal. The sanction applies to both the investigator and the sponsor (company or other) when this type of practice is organised or continued after its discovery.

153

Article 15 of the French medical deontology code says that the physician's duty is to control the consistency of and rationale for the research projects in which he is involved and to check the objectivity of their conclusions. It is not the role of the sponsor to guarantee the morality of an investigator asked to participate in a clinical trial.

The general role of professional councils such as the *Ordre des Médecins* or *Ordre des Pharmaciens*, particularly for industrial pharmacists, is to defend the honour, integrity, and independence of these two professions. Internal disciplinary structures, aim (along with other standards of reference and for other reasons than the civil or the criminal law) for a disciplinary sanction at the worst or, preferably, the prevention of misconduct. This system is difficult to mobilise, especially when the investigator involved is working for the public health service.

Afssaps is also in charge of inspection visits, either as a routine exercise or for cause when fraud is suspected. The inspection team could be helped, when necessary, by other bodies serving more general aspects concerning irregularities, infringements, or repression of fraud.

Given the numerous possible sources of fraud the approach to prevention must be global, taking into account all aspects and all potential perpetrators (see Figure 12.1).

Types of fraud

Whether fraud occurs within the industry itself or at a clinical investigation centre, the types of fraud are the same in France as in other (European) countries. The difficulty of discovery varies, depending upon the possible existence of a whistleblower, the original involvement of the Afssaps, the type of data (modification of a date, clinical parameter or diagnostic procedure, inclusion criteria), and the presence of elements for comparison (for example, sequential events in a single centre, experience of other centres in multicentre studies, etc.). Some frauds involve only a single occurrence (acute fraud), and can be compared at any time with another occurrence preceding the trial. Other cases are more difficult to detect, since they comprise a series of frauds (chronic fraud), each of which may be individually plausible. This type of fraud requires a considerable effort to discover, as does dissimulation or the suppression of data. Discovery of a fraud requires comparison of all available data by comparing documents or a statistical approach.[5–6]

Source documents are an essential reference. Nevertheless, the information necessary for the detection of fraud is not always available in the trial source documents, and it is frequently necessary to have access to the patient's full medical file or the patient him/herself. In some cases this may lead to conflicts between the obligation for medical secrecy and the requirements of the manufacturer or the public authorities. To avoid this type of conflict, the notion of shared secrecy must be accepted by all parties, and officially integrated into the investigator contract and patient informed consent form. This is now possible in France but unfortunately not always elsewhere in Europe.

Other aspects of the typology – the falsification of data, the concealment of data, and the creation of data are considered elsewhere in this book. Nevertheless, falsifications relating to informed consent must be considered separately. These may involve scientific misconduct (for example, absence of informed consent signed by healthy subjects or patients), or real fraud (for example, creation of false consent forms). Informed consent is a basic premise for the protection of patients and is extensively described in official good clinical practice texts. According to French law on biomedical research, the absence of signed consent forms after the study subjects have been given full information about a study, could lead to legal penalties.

Management of fraud

France and most European countries have been strangely absent from the debate concerning management and official sanction of individual cases of fraud, whatever the field of research. This is due both to a tendency of the

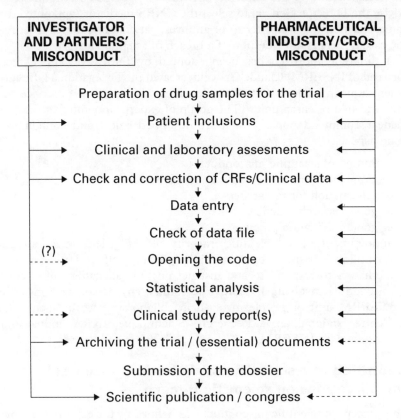

Figure 12.1 Possible times and implications of fraud in clinical trails on medicinal products.

countries to hide such problems, and to the absence of precise and well-codified rules, and it is true for both biomedical research and for clinical trials on medicinal products. Nevertheless, like many US and European research institutions, the principal medical body in France, INSERM, has implemented procedures to respond to allegations of scientific misconduct. This part of the chapter is based on recommendations on scientific integrity, made in 1998 by an INSERM group of experts[7–8] and on papers by the Délégation à l'Intégrité Scientifique (Office of Scientific Integrity) and its head, Déléguée Général Martine Bungener.[9]

INSERM is a French national institute in charge of research in biomedical and health fields. It includes more than 260 units and 9500 people, one third being directly employed by the Institute. For comparison, the Centre National de la Recherche Scientifique (CNRS), has a committee for scientific ethics, Comité d' Éthique pour les Sciences (COMETS), created in 1994, which has a consultative capacity concerning "good scientific practice" and the rules relating to research deontology, such as fraud, capture of scientific results, and plagiarism. Individual situations are the responsibility of the Director General but COMETS is requested to advise the Director General to select the CNRS mediator (appointed for a three-year non-renewable term) or an investigational committee to oversee the case if there is any question of a breach of scientific integrity.

A different approach has been adopted by INSERM. The Director General of INSERM, Claude Griscelli, created the Délégation à l' Intégrité Scientifique in January 1999 after allegations of fraud, in 1997, concerning the head of a research unit.[10] The group of experts appointed at that time made recommendations,[7] which are described below and contain three main aspects:

- definition of scientific misconduct
- recommendations on preventive actions based on:
  - information for researchers
  - good research practice
  - good publication practice
- appointment of a "scientific integrity officer" (délégué à l'intégrité scientifique) assisted by a multidisciplinary staff and nine regional mediators to respond to and instruct possible allegations of scientific misconduct involving INSERM personnel, any person working in an INSERM unit or people involved in collaborative work (such as the Centre National de la Recherche Scientifique, INRA, industry) or contract with INSERM.

Definition of a scientific misbehaviour – general considerations on scientific integrity

The concept of scientific misconduct was defined by the experts as follows: "Scientific misconduct can vary in its seriousness, from insufficient rigor in collecting or presenting data through the deliberate intention to falsify scientific findings or the conditions under which the data were gathered, which constitutes fraud." Even if misconduct does not result from a wilful act, it reveals incompetence that must be analysed and dealt with.

Treatment of such misconduct must be appropriate to its gravity, either by establishing preventive procedures to avoid minor violations or by disciplinary procedures in cases of serious misconduct.

The UK Medical Research Council, on the other hand, defines[11] "scientific integrity ... concerned with being true to the vocation of science and not engaging in plagiarism, selection, enhancement or fabrication of results." This difference in the definition and approach of the question emphasises the difference between the British and French cultures in handling the problem of scientific misconduct.

Recommendations

Advocating a preventive strategy

The INSERM report stresses the importance of preventive steps by:

- keeping researchers informed (young scientists, recently appointed research unit heads)
- the promotion of good research and clinical practice.

In France, the INSERM units involved in clinical trials on medicinal products, comply with the legal requirements (French law on biomedical research and notification of clinical trials to Afssaps) and conform to good clinical practice, subsequently ensuring not only the protection of study subjects but also the quality and reliability of data.

However, the more fundamental type of biomedical research does not comply sufficiently with good laboratory practice. For this reason, INSERM has introduced the systematic use of *research notebooks*, that could be replaced in certain cases by a collection of source documents for clinical data or any form particular to a given discipline (human or social sciences).

This approach is crucial to scientific ethics. All research documents and results (research notebooks) are the property of INSERM and must be archived for 10 years or sent to the INSERM main office when a unit is closed. All contracts between INSERM and a partner, institutions, or industry must show compliance with good laboratory practice and use laboratory notebooks.

A further preventative step is the promotion of ethical guidelines for authorship practices and scientific assessment. Too many factors encourage gift authorship in articles:

- pressure to publish
- encouragement by scientific assessors or reviewers from top ranking journals
- irrational request for top scientific publications for selection/ appointment of hospital practitioners.

INSERM has an Ethical Forum, which is the successor of the previous Ethics Committee; this latter has become the "Comité Consultatif National d'Ethique pour les Sciences de la Vie et de la Santé" (National Advisory Ethics Committee for the Life Sciences and Health). INSERM is intending to publish a document on "good authorship and publication practice".

Implementation of a Délégation à l' Intégrité Scientifique to respond to allegations of fraud

The recommendations of the INSERM experts concerning the allegations of fraud/misconduct are inspired by the systems existing in Germany, the UK, and the USA, and are adapted to the INSERM culture and context.

The aim of the Délégation (its head and mediators) is not only to look at the genesis of the problems that could lead to the development of misconduct but also to propose the most suitable steps to prevent it. There are four separate procedures:

- The *instruction phases* following an allegation of scientific misconduct (instructed by the Délégation, regional mediators, and committees) are separated from the *discipline phase*, which is driven by the INSERM Director General in case of proven fault.
- The three sequential stages must be confidential and instructors should establish whether there is a real fault, its seriousness, and the person(s) responsible.
  - *Stage 1* follows an allegation, accepted only in writing, looks at a local solution decided by the Director General after a suggestion of the regional mediator, and after, if necessary, an interview by Délégation head.
  - *Stage 2* occurs after failure of the previous stage. The Director General appoints experts, with no conflict of interest, in the same field of research, to become the "*committee of enquiry*". The committee sends its conclusions to the Director General, who decides on the consequences.
  - *Stage 3* is a formal investigation by an "*Investigation Committee*" appointed by the Director General and may include foreign experts. Only the Director General is allowed to communicate on the case.
- *Enquiry outcome*
  If a fault is proved, disciplinary or legal measures are taken by the Director General, depending on the importance and the level (individual sanction, closure of the unit). If the fault is not proved, the reputation of the involved person/people needs to be re-established, and necessary sanctions should be taken against the whistleblower in case of defamation.
- *Délégation's annual report*
  The head of the Délégation Générale must provide an annual report to INSERM. This report should contain anonymous statistical data that

should help improve good scientific practice guidelines, in order to protect scientific integrity and avoid fraud and misconduct.

Today INSERM has its own good science practice procedures and its own quality assurance system. These procedures against scientific misconduct are adapted from those of other countries. However, the institution would welcome a European initiative to harmonise good scientific practice in order to prevent or handle cases of fraud. The coordinating organisation could be the European Science Foundation (ESF).

Clinical research on medicinal products

In terms of pharmaceuticals, Europe is said to be divided into two zones: North and South. The North would appear to have a far better reputation and expertise in terms of discovery, development, registration, and manufacture of pharmaceuticals. As in other areas, France finds herself midway between the two as an observer; this is a privileged, intermediate position. Whilst no country is exempt from the risk of fraud in medical research, today it is predominantly the English-speaking and Nordic countries who have established procedures for dealing with this problem. There have been widely publicised cases with appropriate sanctions imposed in Australia, Canada, Nordic countries, the UK, and the USA (open door policy). Even countries such as Japan, traditionally considered to be safe from such abuses for cultural reasons, have recently suffered several scandals involving clinical research.

Management of this problem is difficult in both the individual member states and at the European level, in view of the principle of subsidiarity and despite common pharmaceutical regulations. Each country's code of public health guarantees a high degree of confidentiality of medical files in view of medical secrecy laws.

Any good clinical practice inspection requested by the European Medicines Evaluation Agency must necessarily go through the national agencies (France in this case), with mutual recognition of inspections carried out locally by the national authorities. Today the US Food and Drug Administration inspectors must carry out their own site visits together with a national inspector.

Despite the early and substantial involvement in the internationalisation of drug development, with the exception of Nordic Countries and the UK, none of the European countries has yet undertaken a thorough review of the problem of scientific misconduct during clinical trials of medicinal products.

Most countries maintain a sort of "black list" of persons guilty of fraud during clinical trials on medicinal products, and their identities are known to the responsible persons, mainly health authorities but also the sponsors. The members of Deutche Gesellschaft für Pharmazeutische Medizin (the German Association of Pharmaceutical Medicine),[12] consider themselves

159

responsible for the integrity of clinical data and have a black list called "Golden Memory" with the names of involved physicians, dates, person detecting/notifying the case, description of the case, and the outcome of fraudulent activity. Some of the physicians have been forced to return any money involved to the sponsor; some have been sentenced by the courts and forced to leave hospitals, and some have received prison sentences. Personal communication between the authorities (inspectors of Länders*, scientists of the Bundesinstitut fur Arzneimittel und Medizinprodukte or BfArM) has also proved to be effective. France is progressing very rapidly in admitting to cases of fraud. Afssaps has discovered cases of fraud after inspection. Even French newspapers have publicly denounced fraud for the first time.[1]

The industry and CROs

Good Clinical Practice and Quality Assurance Systems with their "Standard Operating Procedures" (SOPs) improve the quality of clinical trials, allowing adequate monitoring. Audits are carried out by the sponsor and his/her representative is frequently the detector or "whistleblower" of the fraud or misconduct. Most pharmaceutical companies or contract research organisations have a specific standard operating procedure on fraud but suspicions of dishonesty are most frequently covered up for fear of adverse publicity or political problems.

The Regulatory Framework and the Health Products Agency (Afssaps)

The new European Directive on clinical trials

To limit our discussion to the clinical trials required for the registration of new drugs, France falls squarely within Northern Europe in terms of recognition of national studies; this is confirmed by the list of the reporting countries for European centralised and mutual recognition procedures leading to European Marketing Authorisation, and of inspections conducted by the Food and Drug Administration for American new drug applications (NDA). The Southern countries have, so far, less experience, notably because of the lengthy administrative procedures required for initiation of clinical trials. The new European Directive on the implementation of good clinical practice in the conduct of clinical trials on medicinal products for human use,[2] approved in December 2000 by the European Parliament and the Council of Ministers and published as Directive 2001/20/EC, will have to be transposed to the national law of each member state. This law does not include all types of clinical research but, when implemented in the different countries, it will modify the regulatory demand for starting clinical trials on medicinal products, demands to authorities and IECs, and implementation of good clinical practice.

*Länders: states constituting the Federal Republic of Germany

Agence Française de Sécurité Sanitaire des Produits de Santé (Afssaps)

The inspection is defined in the ICH good clinical practice text as:

"The act by a regulatory authority(ies) of conducting an official review of documents, facilities, records, and any other resources that are deemed by regulatory authority(ies) to be related to the clinical trial and that may be located at the site of the trial, at the sponsor and/or contract research organisation's (CRO's) facilities, or at other establishments deemed appropriate by the regulatory authority(ies)."

This part of the chapter is based on a presentation made by Pierre-Henry Berthoye, head of preclinical/clinical inspection of Afssaps and documents provided to the authors by him.[13,14]

The French agency has inspectors (physicians or pharmacists) among its members. They are in charge of compliance by industry, contract research organisations, or any type of sponsors, with the French legal requirements concerning human health products (medicinal products, medical devices, blood derivatives, etc.). French public health inspectors and Afssaps inspectors must ensure compliance with regulatory texts. In the case of scientific misconduct by a physician, the Conseil Régional de l'Ordre des Médecins (Regional Medical Council) can be involved.

The French inspection system of clinical data is national and independent but closely linked to the EMEA inspection unit. The latter coordinates national inspections only for European reasons or in terms of harmonisation of procedures and tools. As each Agency of the European member states, the European Agency for the Evaluation of Medicine (EMEA) has to ensure:

- the protection of persons involved in clinical trials;
- that clinical data collected in order to evaluate the efficacy/efficiency and safety of medicinal products are reliable and of good quality.

At Afssaps, mission statements are given to the non-clinical/clinical inspection department by the Direction de l'Inspection des Essais, either on its own or at the request of the Evaluation Direction of Afssaps, or of EMEA for European procedures of Applications for Marketing Authorisations.

At any time during the life of a medicinal product, the selection of a clinical study is decided by the following criteria:

- at random according to the type of studies (phases, size, regulatory, or epidemiological importance);
- for a specific reason or cause, including one or more of the following items:
  - characteristics of the product and sponsor
  - type of study and study population

- profile of the investigator, team and centre
- complaint of a patient, existence of a whistleblower (person, association, competitor).

For a clinical study to be included in Applications dossier, the evaluation team of Afssaps or EMEA makes a request during a national or European procedure (centralised on mutual recognition) in order to control the quality and reliability of clinical data. The selection is decided according to the above criteria. Specific reasons for selection include: control of the so-called pivotal/essential studies; clinical results (efficacy and/or safety) that differ from similar products; and incoherent data or missing information in the clinical study report.

Conduct of inspections

The French Public Health Code defines the conditions of inspections that are a part of the Afssaps mission. More specifically:

- article L209-3 deals with the the control of compliance with the Code's Livre II bis;
- article L793-10 concerns the appointment of Afssaps inspectors and the exercise of their missions;
- article L795 I/II defines the type of accessible sites in the missions of inspectors;
- article L795 III defines the type and list of documents that must be at the disposal of inspectors, the physician inspectors being the only ones to have the access to clinical data, including patients without breaking medical confidentiality, in order to achieve their mission in the respect of Article 226-13 of the penal code.

Inspection report

The information collected during an inspection by Afssaps inspectors is summarised in a report and transmitted to the Director General of Afssaps. This report is sent to the head of the centre or the sponsor that has been inspected, a legal time frame of 15 days being given for comments or answer.

At the request of the non-clinical/clinical inspection department of Afssaps, a system of markers/triggers for the inspection of clinical studies is under development in Europe, in connection with EMEA and national agencies. The introduction of certain parameters will facilitate the control of clinical data by inspectors working in Europe. This common tool will allow the inspection teams of the member states or others (for example, CADREAC (Collaboration Agreement between Drug Regulatory Authorities in European Union and Associated Countries)), after a common training, to work on harmonised standards, whatever the country where the study was performed.

Clinical research on medicinal products

Sponsor and allegation for or suspicion of fraud

In case of suspicion or detection of misconduct by a representative of the sponsor (hospital, industry, contract research organisations, or other), France has no specific system dealing with fraud, besides the disciplinary and judicial ones, which could emanate from Afssaps. Each of the 15 member states has its own jurisdiction and its own general legal texts, and, with the exception of disciplinary procedures for physicians or pharmacists, clinical research fraud falls within the overall judicial framework for fraud as soon as a complaint has been filed.

Implications for the investigator or other member of the team

Today, any person discovering a case of fraud in France has to consider that the damages may exceed the limits of the contract between the investigator and the sponsor, or that this fraud may cause further damage (registration files, licensing agreements, public health problems, etc.).

Three types of procedures can start in France if fraud is discovered (for example, following an inspection by Afssaps) and a complaint is submitted to a local "Procureur de la République" (Public Prosecution): disciplinary procedures, civil court cases, and criminal court cases. If fraud results in serious damage, judicial recourse can be sought:

- Disciplinary procedures
  Professional societies can take into account any action which affects the collective interest of doctors, including any dishonourable or disreputable acts. In the case of suspected fraud, the French *Ordre des Médecins*, can initiate disciplinary proceedings with potential sanctions ranging up to loss of licence for non-hospital physicians. If the physician works for the public hospital service, the competent administrative authorities (Director of Hospital, Minister of Health) can receive complaints from the sponsor. The punishment may range from censure to dismissal.

- Civil procedures
  The investigator and the sponsor sign a contract involving payment in exchange for acceptance of scientific (protocol), regulatory (good clinical practice), and time constraints. In the case of demonstrated fraud, the judge can set the amount of reparations as a function of the damage done, confirmed by a new expertise (for example, audit) and taking into account whether the repercussions of the fraud were such as to impede proper conduct of the clinical research. However, fraud still constitutes a major problem for the whistleblower. Official procedures leading to sanctions cause problems in France as in

most member states for the sponsor, the investigator, and even health authorities.

- Criminal procedures
  Criminal law sets penalties for fraud, and complaint by the sponsor or the health authorities leads to the initiation of an investigation, which can include the participation of outside experts. In France, in the case of proved fraud, a physician working in the public hospital sector generally incurs more severe sanctions (fines and/or imprisonment) than would be applied to non-hospital personnel.

Fraud by the sponsor

Still harder to detect than fraud by investigators is fraud committed by a manufacturer. This may lead to the invalidation of all or part of a registration file following inspection by the health authorities.

Current situation for clinical trials on medicinal products

Number of Afssaps inspections[14]

From May 1995 to November 2000, the non-clinical/clinical department of Afssaps has performed 199 inspections, referring to clinical trials on medicinal products.

Afssaps findings

The authorities can bring criminal charges against the responsible person within the company, since fraud and forgery are generally punished by imprisonment and/or fines. Disciplinary procedures may also be initiated against any physicians or pharmacists involved. Among the 160 inspections performed between May 1995 and December 1999, 12 allegations of scientific misconduct or fraud were transmitted to the "Public Prosecutor" of the region where the centre in question was located; 10 involved clinical investigators from the private sector and the two others involved manufacturers. The reasons were:

- Refusal of inspection: 1 case
- Falsification of data, use of false data with or without a "risk to others": 10 cases
- Illegal practice of pharmacy (Livre V of CSP*): 1 case
- Non-compliance with Livre II bis of CSP: 1 case

So far no case has been referred to the Ordre des Médecins.

*CSP: Code de la Santé Publique (Code of Public Health)

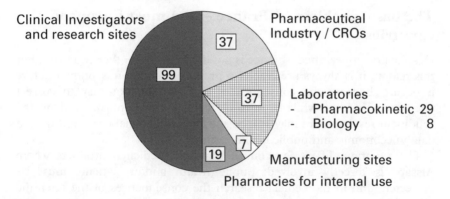

Figure 12.2   Number and distribution of clinical inspections (categories and sites) for clinical studies on medicinal products for human use Agence Française de Sécurité Sanitaire des Produits de Santé – Afssaps.

If we compare the Afssaps experience to the international experience, especially that of the US Food and Drug Administration, the types of findings and scientific misconduct are similar.

Research institutes and scientific misconduct

Research projects

The French experience has been limited up to now and, with a few exceptions[12] allegations of fraud or scientific misconduct have not been officially made in organisations such as the Centre National de la Recherche Scientifique, INSERM or INRA. Since its creation the INSERM office of integrity has had to take care of some allegations of misconduct or conflicts (18 cases in 1999, 25 cases in 2000). Most of these cases were due to internal conflict, mainly about authorship and publications, and not relating to possible misconduct. All the dossiers were started by regional mediators and handled afterwards by the Déléguée à l'Intégrité Scientifique. During this two-year period, the number of allegations was much less than expected by INSERM. Only three committees have had to be set up to interview involved people at the INSERM office of integrity in Paris, following an initial attempt by the regional mediator to solve the problem. One whistleblower put forward one allegation, but the accused person was cleared without prejudice.

If one refers to the US experience,[15] the types of fraud or misconduct appear under the following items:

- fabrication of data
- falsification of results
- plagiarism.

INSERM experience is not so far the same.

The basic problem in France – and most European countries

Despite first appearances, France is not different from other countries. For this reason, it is always preferable to prevent scientific misconduct before it occurs, because the consequences of fraud are not easy to correct afterwards. Indeed, while *a posteriori* control can confirm or deny the validity of results, there may still be substantial financial costs and wasted data in economic and public health terms.

The situation differs for clinical trials on medicinal products where Afssaps is directly involved; public health and/or patients must be protected, and in biomedical research the consequences of the scientific misconduct vary enormously with the project and research domain. However, the basic principle should be the same: ethics in science, good clinical/research practices, and proper training should be developed in France or in Europe as a whole. Whilst all countries have legislation on fraud, this has never prevented its occurrence. In clinical research on medicines, good clinical practice procedures are the only "official" texts that cover this problem and, once fraud is suspected or proved, no sanction is specified except a few lines in the French law on biomedical research, and the civil and criminal codes. Within companies, the standard operating procedures, based upon good clinical practice and drafted by the interested parties with the support of quality assurance and audit department, serve as a basis for prevention. Nevertheless, they are generally written for monitoring outside activities, and few companies have systematic procedures for detecting internal fraud. Similarly, investigators and public bodies generally have no procedures available to monitor fraud, with the exception of INSERM, which now has its own good research practice.

Fraud can be prevented in part by education and also by telling the proposed investigators during prestudy investigator meetings that the study will be monitored during regular periodic visits either by sponsor audit or by official inspection.

The need for a neutral, independent, and confidential approach

We believe that the organisations representing the various partners in France, notably the public health authorities or national research institutions (for example, INSERM) responsible for clinical research, should establish a "charter" concerning fraud and official guidelines to detect fraud at every step. This could include the bases for procedures not only to prevent fraud by the investigators or the sponsors, but also to manage cases of suspected fraud, including sanctions or penalties for the perpetrator. Each company, sponsor, or institution should also draft its own operating procedures for the monitoring of fraud and misconduct according to its own activity and culture.

Since fraud has several possible origins, it would appear desirable first to develop an administrative structure that would be independent of all parties, but where the scientific community would be represented. This independence is needed to maintain impartiality, and would avoid any party bringing the complaint too early to activate major judicial mechanisms that could eventually harm not only the perpetrator of the fraud but also the innocent party.

Monitoring fraud must take into account various constraints: during the investigation, all persons and companies must be treated with respect and protected from adverse publicity. The French so-called "présomption d'innocence" of the person and confidentiality should be guaranteed. However, within these limits, the investigation must be unconstrained. Once the problem has been dealt with, the information should not be made freely available to the public, but should be limited to the regulatory authorities, if the fraud concerns a medicinal product currently marketed, under development, or under registration, on to the head of public research institutions such as INSERM or the Centre Nationale de la Recherche Scientifique, and when appropriate, to the judicial authorities. Complaints can also be brought by individuals, companies, the health authorities (Afssaps-aps), or public institutions.

The file constituting the elements of proof or presumption should always be provided by the party making the complaint (sponsor, investigator, patient, or individual whistleblowers). This document should be as complete as possible, and it may be necessary to include reports from persons other than those directly involved in the study, as well as external auditors.

A French National Committee for Research Integrity after a European model

A European code of practice developed with the support of a European body (for example, European Science Foundation) would help member states, including France, to establish their own system. This harmonised model of a national committee[15] concerning scientific integrity should subsequently be adapted to the culture of each country and the type of research. It could include a common definition of fraud and misconduct; a framework for good science practice, ethics in sciences, guidelines and procedures on different items; it should also describe the activities, composition, functioning of a committee dealing with the allegations of fraud and misconduct. The Nordic model,[16] which is the convergence of procedures of the four Nordic countries, would be a good basis. It would seem preferable that this national committee should function as an aid to the plaintiff, maintaining a purely consultative role.

An educational programme on ethics in science and good research practice should be a priority for the European countries who have not so far addressed this question. France is among these countries.

167

Conclusion

Fraud has always existed and may occur in any human activity. Fraud in clinical research, whether or not pharmaceutical, poses special ethical problems in view of medical and public health issues. There are no European texts specifically devoted to the control of fraud in basic medical research. For clinical research on drugs the new European Directive on Clinical Trials[2] will help to implement the ICH good clinical practice text, in order to protect subjects involved in medical research, as well as to provide high quality, credible data. Fraud itself is not mentioned, but is present in the quality assurance system of the industry with its standard operating procedures, especially in the specific procedure on fraud.

In most European countries, wilful misconduct is not properly handled in the absence of clearly codified regulations; the exceptions are the Nordic countries and UK, which have two different models. The establishment of a European model with a pan-European approach including *ad hoc* committees for each member state of the European Union, including France, should allow us to arrive at a solution for national institutions and health authorities (for example, Afssaps for France). Nevertheless, *prevention is far better than cure*, so:

- University courses concerning the appropriate legal and ethical aspects should be included in the training of research workers (physicians, dentists, pharmacists).
- A more precise legislative framework for dealing with fraud should be developed.
- A professional organisation (committee or association) should be set up in each country, taking into account the general legal framework of fraud prevention.

References

1 Le médecin fournissait trop de cobayes, France – *Soir*, (daily newspaper), Friday 15 December 2000.
2 European Parliament and Council Directive, 2001/20/EC, relating to the implementation of good clinical practice in the conduct of clinical trials on medicinal products for human use.
3 Note for guidance on good clinical practice (CPMP/ICH/135/95).
4 Lock SP, Wells FO eds. *Fraud and Misconduct in Medical Research, Second edition* London: BMJ Publishing Group, 1996.
5 Association of the British Pharmaceutical Industry. *Statistical methods in the investigation of fraud* London: ABPI, 1993.
6 Buyse M, George SL, Evans S *et al*. The role of biostatistics in the prevention, detection and treatment of fraud in clinical trials. *Control Clin Trials* 2000;**21**:415–27.
7 Recommandations du groupe de travailde la Mission de réflexion sur l'intégrité scientifique, actualités, *bulletin de l'institut national de la santé et de la recherche médicale*, 1998,**162**:6–9.
8 Chuat JC. INSERM, délégation à l'intégrité scientifique, personal communication.
9 Bungener M. Procedures for inquiring into Allegations of Scientific Misconduct at INSERM. In: Plehn G, ed. *Ethics of Research, Max Planck Forum 2*, Munich: Max Planck Publishers, 1999.

10 *Le Monde* (daily newspaper) 3 articles on a Rennes INSERM unit.
Le Hir P, Le géne de l'obésité à l'épreuve du soupçon, 22 April 1988.
Brun J-P, Lenfant J, Pourquoi taire unr fraude scientifique? 18 July 1998.
Augereau J-F, L'unité de Rennes sur l'obésité fermée par l'INSERM 29 July 1998.
11 Leech DH. Guaranteeing Good Science Practice in the UK. In: Plehn G, ed. *Max Planck Fourm 2*. Munich: Max Planck Publishers, 1999.
12 Husson JM, Bogaievsky Y, Hvidberg E, Schwarz J, Chadha D, Fraud in clinical research on medicines in the European Union: facts and proposals. In: Lock SP, Wells FO, eds, *Fraud and Misconduct in Medical Research, second edition*. London: BMJ Publishing Group, 1996.
13 Berthoye PH. Eléments pouvant motiver une inspection, Eléments pouvant invalider un essai clinique Meeting on Intégrité et authenticité des données dans la recherche clinique: buts, moyens et conséquences des inspections des essais cliniques, Paris, 20 January 2000.
14 Berthoye PH.: personal communication on Afssaps inspêction figures, with the authorisation of Afssaps.
15 Smith R. The need for a national body for research misconduct. Nothing less will reassure the public, Editorial. *BMJ*, 1998;**316**:1686–7.
16 Riis P. Misconduct in clinical research: The Scandinavian experience and actions for prevention. *Acta Oncologica*, 1999;**38**:89–92.

PART IV
ETHICS AND STATISTICS

13: The role of research ethics committees

JENNIFER BLUNT

Do research ethics committees (RECs) have a role in the detection of misconduct in medical research? This chapter describes how research ethics committees work, suggesting how the system of rigorous ethical review can provide a culture in which it is more difficult for research misconduct to flourish. It demonstrates how research ethics committee review fits with the conclusions of the joint consensus conference on misconduct in biomedical research,[1] with the Committee on Publication Ethics (COPE) guidelines[2] on good publication practice, and research governance in the NHS.[3]

History

At the turn of the 20th century, attention has focused again on research ethics committees. A series of enquiries, including those in Liverpool and North Staffordshire, have highlighted the system whereby research is regulated.[4] This is not new. There have been waves of interest worldwide over the past fifty years in medical research and its regulation, and cases of malpractice have been revealed.

There was widespread horror at Nazi doctors' experiments, which were revealed in the post-war Nuremberg trials in 1947.[5] This led to the Nuremberg Code, which set out principles for the conducting of experiments on humans and which focused on the need for informed consent and a favourable risk:benefit ratio. These principles were later subsumed into the Declaration of Helsinki, 1964,[6] the original version of which related to physicians conducting research on patients and the need for an independent review. It also drew a distinction between therapeutic research for the benefit of treating individual patients, and non-therapeutic research designed to benefit the population at large and where benefit to the individual patient is unlikely.

In 1962 in the USA, it was discovered[7] that many women taking thalidomide during pregnancy had not been told that it was an experimental drug. Unethical clinical research studies were revealed by the American anaesthetist, Henry Beecher, in 1966, and subsequently by the London physician, Maurice Pappworth. In 1972 the Tuskegee Syphilis study in Alabama 1932–1972 showed that 400 African Americans had been denied treatment to demonstrate the natural course of the disease. This ignoble chapter in the history of American public health was finally closed in May 1997, when President Clinton made a public apology to the eight remaining survivors of the study. As a result of these and other research scandals, the US Congress set up a Commission, which issued the Belmont report in 1979. This report provided broad ethical principles, which focused on informed consent, a favourable risk : benefit ratio, and the need to ensure that vulnerable populations are not targeted for risky research.[8] Institutional Review Boards were also set up to review all federally funded research. In the US, controls have been introduced through legislation.

In New Zealand the cervical cancer "trial" was an experimental research programme, where a group of women with carcinoma *in situ* of the cervix had apparently been left untreated or inadequately treated for varying lengths of time. It was the subject of the Cartwright Report, which led to legal regulations governing both research and medical practice.[9]

In the UK, the first official moves began in 1967, when the Royal College of Physicians recommended that clinical research investigations should be subject to ethical review.[10] During this period other guidelines followed from the Royal Colleges, the Medical Research Council, the Association of British Pharmaceutical Industry, and the Department of Health, when local research ethics committees (RECs) were established in 1991 under HSG(91)5, and multicentre research ethics committees in 1997 under HSG(97)23.[11,12] These guidelines evolved gradually, yet are still only guidelines in a country where control of research on animals is very strictly regulated. Although there were recommendations by Neuberger in 1992 for statutory regulation in the UK,[6] there is still no legislation relating expressly to RECs, although, once RECs constitute themselves and review research proposals, they take on legal duties.

Meanwhile, the European Community was moving towards legislation to regulate trials involving medicinal products; practice in the UK is influenced by such European initiatives. The European guidelines, commonly known as "Good Clinical Practice",[13] implemented in the UK in 1991, required clinical trials in general practice to be submitted to RECs for review, for the first time. Further requirements under the International Committee on Harmonisation[14] were issued in 1996. Currently the definitive European Clinical Trials Directive is likely to have far-reaching implications for ethical review in the UK; this Directive could be incorporated into UK law probably in 2003.

Thus, currently in the UK, research is regulated by RECs, which have two major responsibilities:

- the welfare and safety of individual research participants;
- the facilitation of good conduct of high quality research that offers benefits to participants, services, and society at large. Unjustified delay to such research is itself unethical.

Revelations of misconduct in biomedical research are usually greeted with shock and surprise. RECs expect the researcher to be honest and upstanding, someone who will conduct the study as approved by the committee and produce reliable data that will add to the body of knowledge on which biomedical decisions might be based. It is, therefore, necessary to look at what constitutes research misconduct before considering ways of tackling it.

Definitions

Fraudulent research was reported frequently throughout the 1990s. Scientific research misconduct and misconduct in medicine is a growing concern among researchers.[1,15,16]

Various definitions of *research misconduct* have been given: they include fabrication, falsification and/or suppression of data, and plagiarism. It may be an intentional act aimed at misleading someone, in general for personal advantage, but there are other inadvertent acts that may have equally important effects on the quality of scientific research. The Consensus Statement suggests that any definition should allow for change and cover the whole range of research misconduct. It provides the following definition: "Behaviour by a researcher, intentional or not, that falls short of good ethical and scientific standards."[1]

Examples

Research misconduct may involve a range of misdemeanours from failure to get ethics committee approval, falsified patient consent and data, to falsified publications. In the last five years the following cases, from various parts of the world, have been reported in the British medical press.

Invented ethics committee approval

A GP in the UK repeatedly forged ethics committee approval letters.[17] A doctor in public health medicine in Bristol backed applications for research grants with forged letters from ethics committees. He also produced bogus *curricula vitae* to secure academic posts.[18] A hospital doctor in Turkey claimed to have obtained approval from the ethics committee of the medical school and written informed consent from all patients; neither claim was true.[19]

Inventions

An American cell biologist was found to have intentionally falsified and fabricated data.[20] Another UK GP submitted the same electrocardiogram for more than one patient.[21] A Spanish doctor was jailed for four years for accepting bribes from a pharmaceutical company manager to fabricate studies of pharmacological follow up.[22] Two German cancer specialists were found to have manipulated data and images in research papers.[23]

The same cancer specialists were also found to have forged and invented data in 47 scientific articles. A breast cancer researcher at the University of Witwatersrand was accused of, and later admitted at an international conference, to misrepresenting results of a clinical trial.[24]

A further GP in the UK was found guilty of falsifying patient consents.[25] Handwriting experts found that the consent forms of a large proportion of patients entered into two trials, by the second GP referred to above, had not been signed by the patients themselves.[21]

Not following protocol as approved

A former professor in respiratory medicine in London was struck off the medical register for trying to persuade a junior colleague to break a blinded trial code, a protocol violation, by using bullying and threatening behaviour.[26]

Who does it?

Research misconduct is committed by general practitioners and hospital and academic doctors, the young and inexperienced, and those at the very top of the profession. Rennie suggests that the bestowal of a scientific or medical degree is not accompanied by a guarantee of honesty.[27] In a review by the US Office of Research Integrity, it was found that half of the biomedical researchers accused of scientific fraud and formally investigated were found guilty of misconduct. These cases of misconduct were mostly of falsification and fabrication of data, but also included plagiarism. Researchers of all grades commit fraud, but the more senior people are, the more likely they are to get away with it: assistant professors seem to attract most allegations of misconduct.[28]

It is very worrying that 36% of medical students said they would be prepared to falsify patient information, plagiarise other people's work, or forge signatures.[1] More recently, the editor of the *British Medical Journal* drew attention to a case of cheating in exams,[29] which was followed by a very large number of electronic responses on the acceptability or otherwise of cheating. It has been argued that scientists must be taught about good and bad research practices and about research ethics, and that, if senior scientists make efforts to become close mentors to their juniors, this will raise standards considerably.[27] That assumes, of course, that mentors are not fraudulent themselves.

Research ethics committee review

This chapter suggests that rigorous ethical review by RECs is a powerful preventative measure in tackling research misconduct. Researchers conducting any research in the NHS are required to submit their proposals to a REC for ethical approval before starting their project. A REC is in a unique position, being the most independent body regulating the ethical conduct of clinical research.[30]

Function of research ethics committees

Research ethics committees provide independent advice to health authorities, participants, researchers, funders, sponsors, care organisations, and professionals on the extent to which proposals for the study comply with recognised ethical standards.[3,11] This advice applies to university staff, who also require REC approval in addition to the university's ethics committee if their work involves the NHS.

The European Directive states that a clinical trial may be undertaken only if the foreseeable risks and inconveniences have been weighed against the expected benefit for the individual trial subject and society, and the rights of the subject to physical and mental integrity, to privacy, and to the protection of the data concerning him are safeguarded.

Composition of research ethics committees

RECs are independent bodies and include members who are non-medical as well as those from the healthcare professions. The committees are not medically dominated, usually less than half of the membership being medically trained. Members reflect a mix of gender, age, and ethnic background, with a broad range of experience sufficient to reconcile the scientific and medical aspects of the research proposal with the welfare of research subjects and broader ethical implications.[11,12]

What is needed in ethical review is careful, rational thinking by groups of people who collectively understand the importance of different moral claims, and who can work constructively together to come to sound and reasonable conclusions.

Scope

Local research ethics committees (LRECs) were set up in 1991[11] and multicentre research ethics committees (MRECs) in 1997[12] to give prior ethical approval to all research in the NHS, including clinical trials; records-based, qualitative, and Heath Services economic research; and surveys, involving individuals, their tissue, or data.[3] They also advise on health-related non-NHS research.

Distribution of duties between MRECs and LRECs

LRECs are responsible for the review of all research in their own geographical areas, except when it is multicentre research. In this instance, MRECs provide independent advice on scientific aspects and general ethics of multicentre research taking place within five or more LREC boundaries, and then LRECs determine the criteria for local acceptability of researchers, site, and subjects.

- *The suitability of a local investigator* could be judged in relation to published guidelines on good clinical practice,[13,14] the volume of current research, and the track record of researchers. It is the responsibility of the pharmaceutical physician and clinical trial monitor

177

to ensure that only reliable investigators are recruited. Companies should reject any potential investigator about whom there are doubts arising from past involvement in a research project.

LRECs should know of an investigator's involvement in concurrent trials.[31] It has been suggested that local investigators could be registered as suitable after an initial screening test; thereafter suitability could be a matter of an administrative checklist. This, however, may not be the most appropriate way to deal with the moral aspects of suitability.

- *The suitability of the site* could be judged by a site visit to determine whether the facilities contain the necessary equipment and experienced support staff to conduct the research. Excellent "hotel" facilities, however, do not necessarily guarantee good research.
- *The suitability of the project* for local participants could be judged by consideration of the current disease patterns, particular social and cultural needs of the local population, and the need to protect patients with rare or "fashionable" conditions from unwarranted scientific curiosity.

Process of ethical review

RECs are required to review research projects for their ethical acceptability. In this process, members should be mindful that:

- they must protect patients and the public against harm from research and against useless studies, which are unethical;[32]
- they should encourage research that will in the long run improve health care and health[32] and facilitate ethically acceptable attempts to identify new and better treatments from which all may potentially benefit.

The fundamental principles of ethics committee review are the same, whether the research in question is a large multicentre study or a smaller scale local investigation, the review should be effective and the process should be efficient. The Briefing Pack for Research Ethics Committee Members[33] sets out structured approach to ethical analysis (Table 13.1).

Table 13.1   Assessment template.

What a research ethics committee looks for	Ethical approach
• Validity of the research	Design
• How important is the research question?	Goal-based
• Can the research answer the question being asked?	
• Welfare of the research subject	Risks/harms
• What will participating in the research involve?	Duty-based
• Are any risks necessary and acceptable?	
• Dignity of the research subject	Consent/confidentiality
• Will consent be sought?	Rights-based
• Will confidentiality be respected?	

> **Box 13.1 Application form: details to be provided by the researcher**
>
> - Details of applicant
> - Details of project
> - Recruitment of subjects
> - Consent
> - Details of interventions
> - Risks and ethical problems
> - Compensation and confidentiality

These principles are translated into practice in the standard application form, model patient information sheet, and consent form used by most research ethics committees (Box 13.1).

From the application form members will then be able to form a view on the points to consider as laid out in HSG(91)5.

Consideration of the protocol

Details of applicant

A *curriculum vitae* is required from the principal applicant. Basic scientists are required to hold honorary NHS contracts in order to have access to patients or their data. Do the skills of the investigator match the subject of the study? Where supervision is appropriate, is it adequate? A figurehead expert could be too busy to provide personal supervision.

Supervision becomes particularly important where students, at whatever level, are carrying out research on NHS patients or their records. Excuses like, "It is only a little blood" or "Only a few questions" or "A quick look at notes", may disguise the fact that patients could simply be the means to serve the ends of the student. Much research undertaken by students on human participants ignores compliance with established conventions, such as the Declaration of Helsinki[6] and other guidelines that are designed to protect those taking part in biomedical research.

Details of project

Researchers should set out their method clearly in this section. Members will consider the importance of the research question, whether the study design can answer the question being asked, and whether the research is necessary. Research that duplicates other work unnecessarily or that is not of sufficient quality to contribute something useful to existing knowledge is in itself unethical.

RECs require scrupulous observance of scientific standards including, where appropriate, the use of sound, accepted statistical techniques to produce reliable and valid data. In a randomised controlled trial, does

179

equipoise exist? Will comparisons be made against comparators and not placebo, as in line with the fifth version of the Declaration of Helsinki?[6] In qualitative research will appropriate, validated tools be used?

Recruitment of subjects

Researchers must show that the selection of participants is fair and appropriate. Sometimes groups are excluded unfairly. Should women of child-bearing potential be involved? Should there be an upper age limit? Must many people with learning disabilities be excluded because of impaired ability to consent? What about the selection of children? About 40% of drugs used to treat children are not licensed for that purpose, because few drug companies are willing to undertake such trials. All sections of the community should be able to benefit from the results of research.

Participants should be recruited through a known intermediary. Direct approaches from a researcher would be a breach of confidentiality. Methods of direct recruitment are currently under scrutiny by RECs.

Consent

Will written consent be sought? Will consent be given freely? Will participants be offered the ability to take part or to refuse/withdraw? There are particular requirements when consent is being sought for the use of tissue or blood in genetic studies, where samples may be stored for a future, unspecified, research purpose. Guidelines from the MRC and Royal College of Pathologists are of relevance.[34-38]

As part of the consent process, would-be participants need full information, clearly expressed and without details that could mislead. Model patient information sheets are now available. Those for genetic studies must acknowledge the participant's right to know or their right not to know. There must be protection of patient data in line with the Data Protection Act 1998, with particular attention to systems for ensuring confidentiality of personal information and the security of these systems.[39] Members will need to know that researchers understand the levels of security between coded and anonymised samples.

Genetic information has great potential in drug development. It is very important in research that involves genetic testing that participants understand the significance of the information generated, its power, predictiveness, and implications for the welfare of other family members. Members will want to know that consent is truly informed, and that issues about storage, confidentiality, privacy, and feedback of information to trial participants have been dealt with adequately.

Details of interventions

Researchers must make clear the risk of possible side effects, whether they are known or unknown. Drug interactions and exclusion criteria have to be considered; a warning about the simultaneous taking of over-the-counter remedies may need to be given. Will there be physical discomfort from invasive techniques, such as repeated venepunctures or endoscopies? Could there be psychological distress from intrusive questionnaires? Will extra visits or travelling be acceptable?

Risks and ethical problems

Researchers need to show that they understand the ethical problems. Answers here will reveal how the health and welfare of those who take part will be affected, including their rights, safety and well-being. Are there any risks to taking part and, if so, are they necessary and/or acceptable? Might the use of databases for recruitment lead to the overresearching of a core group of patients with specific diseases? Participants should be told what alternatives exist and what will happen at the end of the trial, and whether trial medication or trial therapy will continue to be available.

Compensation and confidentiality

The *indemnity* for the study must be appropriate, and evidence must be furnished. This should be in keeping with the Association of British Pharmaceutical Industry guidelines on no-fault compensation, NHS indemnity or university insurance cover for ethically approved studies. Participants who are NHS patients may receive reimbursement of expenses but not for taking part in studies. Any form of inducement is unacceptable.

Will *confidentiality* be respected? Most information about people drawn from interviews, medical records, scientific tests, and surveys is confidential. Members will want to know how researchers will collect, store, and process confidential information in line with recent guidelines.[39] They need to know that researchers have ensured that their work is consistent with the law and that participants have agreed at the outset what information about them will be used.

The process of ethical review when there is no local researcher

This applies particularly to epidemiological and health services research. In November 2000, an operational modification of the MREC system was introduced to cover the situation where there is no need for a local researcher and hence no need for local scrutiny by an LREC.[40] It will use the technical cooperation of the patient's local clinician without designating the clinician as a local researcher.

Hence researchers need to undergo close scrutiny in the process of ethical review.

Post-approval duties

Post-approval duties of RECs are limited to requiring the submission of an annual progress report, amendments, and reports of adverse events.[11] Despite calls[6,10] for RECs to follow up the studies that they approve, RECs in the UK do not have a role in monitoring studies as they proceed. The principal investigator, the research sponsor, and the care organisation, and not the research ethics committee, are responsible for ensuring that a study

181

follows the agreed protocol and for monitoring its progress.[3] Arrangements exist in Canada and Italy for such monitoring.

RECs in the UK are advisory bodies. They must maintain independence when formulating their advice on the ethics of the proposed research in order that their advice is seen to be impartial. They are managerially independent of NHS Trust R&D structures.[3] They are not legal entities in themselves, are not financed to take on monitoring duties, and have no executive function.

Commercially sponsored studies are closely monitored by project managers and clinical research associates working to well-defined standard operating procedures. The MRC have set up trial steering committees to oversee the scientific acceptability and the overall conduct of their trials with an independent data monitoring and ethics committee to analyse the data.[35] Other funding organisations are following the same model with a trial committee to monitor the trial progress and implement any recommendations made by the independent data monitoring committee. Such committees regularly review the unblinded data and primary outcome measures and can recommend the early termination of studies, if necessary.

Links with COPE guidelines consensus statement/ research governance framework

Since 1997 there have been three major initiatives in which research misconduct has been tackled. The Committee on Publication Ethics (COPE)[2] was formed by a group of medical editors, who have produced guidelines on good publication practice (see Chapter 18). A Joint Consensus Conference on Misconduct in Biomedical Research in Edinburgh in 1999[1] agreed a statement on research misconduct and the promotion of good research. Most recently, the Department of Health issued a consultation draft research governance framework for health and social care.[3]

COPE

Intellectual honesty should be actively encouraged in all medical and scientific courses of study, used to inform publication ethics, and prevent misconduct. It is with that in mind that these guidelines have been produced. Good research should be well justified, well planned, appropriately designed, and ethically approved. To conduct research to a lower standard may constitute misconduct.

Consensus statement

Patients benefit not only from good quality care but also from good scientific research. We all expect high standards of scientific and medical research practice. The integrity, probity, skill, and trustworthiness of scientific and medical researchers are essential if public confidence is to be assured. In the design of biomedical and healthcare research, public participation is essential.[1]

Research governance framework

The Government is committed to enhancing the contribution of research to health and social care, and the partnership between services and science. The public has a right to expect high standards (scientific, ethical, and financial), transparent decision-making processes, clear allocation of responsibilities, and robust monitoring arrangements. A quality research culture is essential for proper governance of health and social care research.[3]

These initiatives agree on the need for:

- a culture of quality, honesty, and integrity in research
- formal ethical approval
- consent and confidentiality
- good research practice
- publication and accessible accounts of research
- appropriate monitoring of progress of studies
- formal supervision of researchers
- systems for managing misconduct
- guidance and training for research ethics committees and for researchers.

The recommendations of the research governance framework were designed to promote excellent quality research and, conversely, to prevent less good practice. This is the task that RECs set out to perform. Their rigorous ethical review is one means whereby research misconduct can be minimised.

Investigation route(s) to take in cases of suspicion

RECs are advisory bodies without executive functions; they are not detective agencies, they are not legal entities in themselves, and they have no authority to investigate suspected or admitted misconduct. Their duty is to bring the matter to the attention of their establishing body – usually the health authority/commission or trust, as directed in HSG(91)5:

Para 3.22
LREC advice not requested or ignored
If it comes to the attention of a committee that research is being carried out, which it has not been asked to consider or which it has considered but its recommendations have been ignored, then the LREC should bring the matter to the attention of its appointing authority, the relevant NHS body and to the appropriate professional body.

Thereafter RECs should cooperate in the investigations led by others. An REC is in a prime position to assist, being probably the only source of comprehensive information about an individual investigator's research activity. RECs have no power to ensure that all research is submitted to them or to stop research that they regard as unethical. They cannot know about research where an investigator is deliberately circumventing ethical review, examples of which are quoted elsewhere in this chapter. They also do not know of studies that the researchers themselves have chosen to regard as audit, which in general does not require ethical approval.

Health research carried out by the NHS in England and Wales must meet new standards designed to protect participants, improve quality, and stop research fraud. The research governance consultative document[3] identifies growing public and professional concern about research misconduct and fraud. It refers to appropriate systems for detecting, investigating, and addressing fraud, along with those with whom they have partnership arrangements. Many bodies already have or are updating their procedures.

Conclusions

Rigorous review by research ethics committees can:

- provide a powerful preventative measure in tackling research misconduct;
- provide a culture in which it is more difficult for research misconduct to flourish;
- help prevent less good research practice and protect patients and the public against harm from research and researchers;
- encourage a culture in which good quality, well-justified, well-planned, and appropriately designed biomedical research can flourish;
- facilitate ethically acceptable attempts to identify new and better treatments from which all may potentially benefit.

References

1 Christie B. Panel needed to combat research fraud. *BMJ* 1999;**319**:1222.
2 Jones J. UK watchdog issues guidelines to combat medical research fraud. *BMJ* 1999; **319**:660–1.
3 Department of Health. *Draft research governance framework for health and social care.* London: DOH, September 2000.
4 NHS Executive. *West Midlands Regional Office report of a review of the research framework in North Staffordshire Hospital NHS Trust.* May 2000.
5 Neuberger J. Ethics and health care. *King's Fund Institute Research Report* 47, 1992.
6 World Medical Association Declaration of Helsinki. *Recommendations guiding physicians in biomedical research involving human subjects.* Adopted by the 18th WMA General Assembly, Helsinki, Finland, June 1964 and amended by the 29th WMA General Assembly, Tokyo, Japan, October 1975; 35th WMA General Assembly, Venice, Italy, October 1983; 41st WMA General Assembly, Hong Kong, September 1989; 48th WMA General Assembly, Somerset West, Republic of South Africa, October 1996; and the 52nd WMA General Assembly, Edinburgh, Scotland, October 2000.
7 Smith T. *Ethics in medical research. A handbook of good practice.* Cambridge: Cambridge University Press, 1999.
8 Emanuel E, Wendler D, Grady C. What makes clinical research ethical? *JAMA* 2000;**283**:2701–11.
9 Paul C. Internal and external morality of medicine: lessons from New Zealand. *BMJ* 2000;**320**:499–503.
10 Royal College of Physicians of London. *Guidelines on the practice of ethics committees in medical research involving human subjects* (2nd edn). London: RCP, 1990; (3rd edn). London: RCP, 1996.
11 Department of Health. *Local research ethics committees.* London: DOH, 1991 HSG(91)5.
12 Department of Health. *Ethics Committee Review of multi-centre research.* London: DOH, 1997 HSG(97)23.
13 Commission of the European Communities; CPMP Working Party on Efficacy of Medicinal Products. *Notes for guidance on good clinical practice for trials on medicinal products in the European Community.* Brussels: European Community, 1991.

14 International Conference on Harmonisation of Technical Requirements for Regulation of Pharmaceuticals for Human Use. *Tripartite guideline for good clinical practice*. Geneva: IFPMA, 1996.

15 Smith R. Time to face up to research misconduct. *BMJ* 1996;**312**:789–90.

16 Farthing MJG. An editor's response to fraudsters. *BMJ* 1998;**316**:1726–33.

17 Carnall D. Doctor struck off for scientific fraud. *BMJ* 1996;**312**:400.

18 Dyer C. Doctor admits research fraud *BMJ* 1998;**316**:645.

19 Horton, R. Retraction: Interferon alfa-2b…in Behçet's disease. *Lancet* 2000;**356**:1292.

20 Dobson R. US research scientist found guilty of fraud. *BMJ* 1999;**319**:1156.

21 Dyer O. GP found guilty of forging trial consent forms. *BMJ* 1998;**317**:1475.

22 Bosch X. Three jailed in bribery and prescription fraud scandal. *BMJ* 1999;**319**:1026.

23 Tuffs A. Fraud investigation concludes that self regulation has failed. *BMJ* 2000;**321**:72.

24 Gottlieb S. Breast cancer researcher accused of serious scientific misconduct. *BMJ* 2000;**320**:398.

25 Dyer C. GP struck off for fraud in drug trials. *BMJ* 1996;**312**:798.

26 Dyer C. London professor struck off for bullying and dishonesty. *BMJ* 1999;**319**:938.

27 Rennie D. An American perspective on research integrity. *BMJ* 1998;**316**:1726–33.

28 Pownall M. Falsifying data is main problem in US research fraud review. *BMJ* 1999;**318**:1164.

29 Smith R. Cheating at medical school. *BMJ* 2000;**321**:398.

30 Blunt J, Savulescu J, Watson AJM. Meeting the challenge facing research ethics committees: some practical suggestions. *BMJ* 1998;**316**:58–61.

31 Royal College of Physicians of London. *Report on fraud and misconduct in medical research*. London: RCP, 1991.

32 Alberti KGMM. Multicentre research ethics committees: has the cure been worse than the disease? *BMJ* 2000;**320**:1157–8.

33 Department of Health. *Briefing pack for research ethics committee members*. London: DOH, 1997.

34 Medical Research Council. *MRC policy and procedure for inquiring into allegations of scientific misconduct*. London: MRC, December 1997 (MRC ethics series).

35 Medical Research Council. *Guidelines for good clinical practice in clinical trials*. MRC, March 1998.

36 Medical Research Council. *Human tissue and biological samples for use in research: MRC interim operational and ethical guidelines*. Consultation November 1999. London: MRC, 1999.

37 Royal College of Pathologists. *Consensus statement of recommended policies for uses of human tissue in research, education and quality control*. London: RCP, 1999.

38 Royal College of Pathologists. *Guidelines for the retention of tissues at post-mortem examination*. London: RCP, March 2000.

39 Medical Research Council. *Personal information in medical research: MRC guidelines*. MRC/55/00. London: MRC, 5 October 2000 (MRC ethics series).

40 Department of Health. *Ethical review of multicentre research in the NHS where there is no local researcher*. London: DOH, November 2000.

14: Statistical aspects of the detection of fraud*

STEPHEN EVANS

Round numbers are always false.
Samuel Johnson

The very use of the word "data" (from the Latin "given") suggests that those who receive data for analysis do so in the spirit of a gift. To question the veracity of data is then to look the gift horse in the mouth. It may be wise, however, to have at least the level of suspicion that the Trojans were advised to have when confronted with their gift horse.

The emphasis in statistical textbooks and training is on analysing the data, assuming they are genuine. Checking the data is sometimes mentioned,[1,2] although this is directed mainly at the possibility of accidental errors rather than at deliberate falsification. Altman notes that, "It is the large errors that can influence statistical analyses."[2] Accidental errors that are large clearly affect the analysis, but alteration or invention of data will be done in a way to attempt to conceal their false nature. The features of these false data will not be the same as ordinary errors. In spite of this, careful use of the best procedures for data checking with some simple extensions will go a long way to detect many instances of fraud. This chapter will outline routine methods for checking data that will help to correct accidental errors as well as the problems that are the target of this book. The accidental errors in data are (one hopes) more frequent than deliberate ones, so that effort expended in checking data will result in better quality reports of medical science even in the absence of attempts to cheat.

The power of modern computer programs for statistical data analysis is a great help with this type of data checking, but also facilitates fabrication of data. More emphasis in the training of statisticians needs to be given to this aspect of data analysis, since a perfect analysis on the wrong data can be much more dangerous than an imperfect analysis of correct data. It has been suggested that statisticians should not publish too much on the methods to detect fraud, since then those wishing to pervert science without being caught will learn how to avoid detection. Whilst this could be

*The author is grateful for comments from Dr P Lachenbruch in revising this chapter.

partially true, there will always be new, as yet unpublished, methods that will be invented by the vigilant statistician to detect invented data.

Types of fraud

Relatively little has been published about the particulars of fraudulent data, so that most statisticians have little or no experience in this field. From what is known we can divide the problems into two major groups:

- data *manipulation* to achieve a desired result or increase the statistical significance of the findings and affect the overall scientific conclusions;
- *invention* of data for non-existent or incomplete cases in clinical studies.

The motives in the first instance are to achieve publication, or to produce results confirming a particular theory, rather than financial considerations. The motives in the second are usually for financial gain. Most of the well known cases of fraud in the UK fall into this category. There are possibly some instances where academics have produced fictitious data to publish a paper or form material for a thesis, but this has been difficult to prove. A particular form of data manipulation is to include those who are ineligible according to the protocol for the study. Similarly it is possible that eligible subjects are excluded. These could be regarded as a separate category. These actions tend to have little effect on the internal validity, but could have an important effect on external validity (generalisability) of the study.

Publication bias is a well known feature of the scientific literature, in which results that are highly statistically significant are more likely to be published than those showing smaller effects. Hence, some fraud is directed at obtaining statistical significance of the results. Several publicised cases of this type have occurred in the USA but they are also known in Europe. This type of fraud tends to occur in academically related research, where career advancement is the ultimate motive. More details of known instances of fraud are given by Lock in Chapter 4 of this volume.

Characteristics of genuine data and their analysis

In biological and especially in medical investigation there is usually considerable variation in any phenomenon studied. A major contribution of statistical methodology is in quantifying variability and in distinguishing random variation from genuine effects. Statistical significance tests (or confidence intervals) are one way of classifying genuine as opposed to spurious effects. The object of most fraud is to demonstrate a "statistically significant" effect that the genuine data would not show.

Most medical research looks for evidence of some effect such as a new treatment for a disease. The effect will be shown by differences between a treated and a control group. In a statistical significance test (or confidence interval), there are three components that are combined to show the strength of the evidence:

- the magnitude of the effect
- the variability of individuals in the study
- the number of individuals studied.

Evidence for the existence of an effect is when the first and third are as large as possible and when the second is as small as possible. Most fraud intended to demonstrate an effect consists of reducing variability and increasing the number of individuals.

In some senses the opposite problem occurs when a study is designed to show the similarity of two treatments. These "equivalence trials", or often in practice, "non-inferiority trials", are particularly vulnerable to invented data. These types of trial have an increasing place in the development of drugs by the pharmaceutical industry. There are ethical pressures to avoid the use of placebos, but the consequence is that introducing a lot of "noise" can make treatments look similar. Increase in individual variability leads to failing to find statistically significant differences, especially if the mean is similar in the two groups, as happens when "noise" is introduced. Invented data can make treatments appear similar, and hence a new product could be licensed on the basis that it is similar to an older product for which there is evidence of efficacy. This can have adverse consequences for public health. Adverse effects could also appear to be similar between treatments if data are invented.

The large amount of variability in genuine data not only makes the use of statistical methods important in medical research, but also tends to be hidden when summary statistics of data are presented. Whenever summaries of data are presented, they should be accompanied by some measure of the variability of the data.

Wherever measurement involves human judgment, even in reading data from an instrument, the data show special features. One of these features is "digit-preference". This is well known in blood pressure, where clinical measurements tend to be recorded to the nearest 5 mmHg or 10 mmHg. Where it is recorded to 5 mmHg, it is still more usual to find values with a last digit of 0 than of 5. In research, measurements may be made to the nearest 2 mmHg.

Another example is in recording babies' birthweights. Figure 14.1 shows an example of data from a large national study done in 1958. In this diagram the weights are shown to the nearest ounce, and it is clear that certain values are much preferred to others. Whole pounds are the most frequent, with half and quarter pounds and two ounces being progressively less "popular", while very few weights are recorded to the nearest ounce. In data measured in the metric system, the preferences are for values recorded to the nearest 500, 250 or 100 grams.

Errors of measurement and of recording occur in all genuine data, and some individuals show an idiosyncratic response. These factors result in

Birthweight distribution

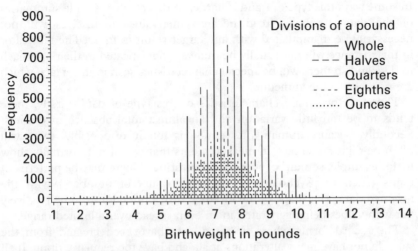

Source – National child development survey

Figure 14.1   Value preference in recording babies' birthweights.

"outliers" occurring in the data. When they are genuine values they should be included in the analysis, but when there is good external evidence that they are errors (for example, age = 142 years) they should be corrected or eliminated. Most effort in data checking is directed towards these values as noted above.

Characteristics of fraudulent data

Manipulated data

Fraudulent manipulation is likely to attempt to show a desired effect by manipulating the data in any or all of the three ways that affect the statistical significance of the results noted above:

- larger differences between groups appear
- variability of results is reduced
- extra data are invented.

The main way is by reducing variability, so that observations that do not "fit" the desired result are deleted or amended. Simple invention of data tends to result in a series of values that are too close to each other. It needs considerable familiarity with the field of study, or the examination of other people's results to be able to recognise this reduced variability.

The number of changes made on original record forms may also be increased when manipulation of the data takes place by changing the record forms.[3]

189

Simple invented data

In some ways this type of fraud is harder to detect when simple summaries of the data are being read because the values themselves will not necessarily be manipulated with any target result in mind. The fabricator in this instance will not usually be quite as sophisticated in their approach to data and so there will be special characteristics seen in the ersatz, which are not seen in the authentic.

There are two main characteristics of this type of data. Firstly, there tends to be too little variation and an almost total absence of outliers. Secondly, because human intervention is totally responsible, there will often be digit preference in measurements that would not normally show it (for example, sodium concentration in urine). There may be patterns of digits (such as psychologically preferred pairs of numbers) with the invented data. The shape of the invented distribution tends to be relatively flat with values being generated in an even spread over a limited range.

The record forms where invented data have been created from the start do not have many alterations at all, and have too regular writing. If all the forms have been completed in the same pen, this may be spotted by those involved in entering or checking the record forms from a clinical trial.

Methods for detecting problems

In some senses the methods for detection of problems are simply an extension of the usual methods for checking data, combined with an awareness of the characteristics shown by altered and fabricated data. There are some purely statistical methods, and some graphical methods, which supplement the numerical ones. Familiarity with the research subject is also important, which will be true from medical investigator and referee, but may not be true for the statistician analysing the data. This knowledge will include a sensitivity to look for relationships that should exist and for the absence of relationships that should not.

Examining data: one variable at a time

The features of fraudulent data such as excessive digit preference or alteration of record forms will not usually be visible to the reader, referee, or editor, but may be detected if looked for by a colleague or statistician processing the raw invented data. Digit preference itself is neither a sensitive nor a specific test of fraud.

Statistical methods

The methods for data checking described in textbooks aimed at medical research such as Altman[2] and Altman et al.[4] are entirely appropriate. However, they have an implicit assumption that the data are genuine; using

190

the presentation methods that they suggest will be a first step in preventing fraud. Checking will usually be needed by centre or investigator, or time period, when the main analysis would not be done in this way.

The guidelines that were previously published in the *BMJ* and that have been updated in Chapters 9 and 10 of Altman *et al.*[4] are particularly pertinent. The use of standard deviations and percentile ranges (such as 25th–75th or 10th–90th) may be helpful. The range itself is focused on the extremes (that are the observations most likely to be in error), and always increases with increasing sample size. It may be helpful in detecting outliers (or their absence), but should not be a substitute for measures such as the standard deviation that can be used for comparative purposes across different studies. If the range of observations is clearly determined, such as lying within 0–100 as a percentage of another measurement that forms a total, it is unlikely to be helpful itself. However, the percentiles can still be quite different in real as opposed to invented data. The range is more popular in the medical literature than it should be, and is often the only measure of variability quoted in published reports.

Original data should be summarised wherever possible rather than only derived variables. A confidence interval or a standard error may allow for the derivation of the standard deviation provided the sample size involved is clear to the reader. Provided this is possible, then constraints on space may allow standard deviations to be omitted, although they can often be included with very little space penalty.

For those with access to the raw data there are a variety of techniques that can be used to detect problems. The variation in the data is a vital component to examine. The kurtosis of a distribution is not often used in ordinary statistical analysis, but can be very helpful, both in scanning for outliers in many variables, and also in looking for data that have too few outliers. Data that are from a uniform distribution can be detected by examination of the kurtosis. It is especially helpful within the context of a large and complex trial in scanning many variables in a large number of centres, separately by treatment group.

Dates are helpful in checking veracity. In some instances, fraudulent data have involved supposed visits to a general practitioner or hospital outpatient clinic on bank holidays or weekends. While not impossible, these are less likely, and where any number of visits are recorded on such dates this constitutes a "signal" of an issue that merits investigation. As with other data, reduced variability in times between visits is a marker of possible problems. Buyse *et al.*[5] give a description of this type of problem in more detail, with an example from Scherrer.[6]

Authors (and editors) should be encouraged to present raw data if possible rather than just summary values, and, where practicable, diagrams that show all the data should also be presented. Bad data tend to lie too close to the centre of the data for their own group. All authors should be ready to send their data, if requested, to an editor so that independent checks may be made on it if necessary.

191

Graphical methods

These are part of statistical science and require careful thought for scientific presentation. The advent of business presentation graphics on personal computers has led to a decline in the quality of published graphs. Inappropriate use of bar graphs for presenting means is a typical example. The use of good graphics is particularly useful when patterns are being sought in data under suspicion.

Some techniques may be used for exploration of data but may not be the best for final communication of the results. An example is the use of the "stem and leaf" plot. This is like a histogram on its side, with the "stem" being the most significant digits, and the "leaves" being the least significant digits. This can be constructed by hand very easily, and many statistical computer programs can produce it. Because it retains all the data, unlike the histogram, which groups the data, the last digit can be seen, and instances of digit preference can be seen clearly. Such a technique showed that doctors did not always use the Hawksley random zero sphygmomanometer in the correct manner.[7] This example itself illustrates that, as with the title of that paper, it is always easier to blame a machine than human failing.

Figure 14.2 shows a stem and leaf plot of blood pressure recorded in another study where, although the measurements were theoretically made to the nearest 2 mmHg, some minor digit preference may be seen.

Stem and leaf plots could be used in publications more than they are, and for further details of their construction see Altman[2] or Bland.[8] If digit preference is suspected, then a histogram of the final digit, or a separate

Depth	Stem	Leaves	Plot of DBP
2	5●	68	
12	6★	0222224444	
16	●	6666	
33	7★	00000022222222444	
(8)	●	66668888	
37	8★	00000022244444	
23	●	666888	
17	9★	000024	
11	●	666	
5	10★	000	
3	●	88	
	11★	4	
	HIGH	118, 140	

Figure 14.2   Stem and leaf plot of diastolic blood pressure. The first two values are 56, 58. Note that there are 21 values ending in zero, while 11 values end in 8. This is only slight digit preference. (The values are not expected to be measured to better than 2 mmHg.)

192

one of the penultimate digit can be helpful. A *chi*-square test for the goodness of fit to a uniform distribution offers a guide as to whether the digit preference is more than random variation. When measurements are made by human reading, such as height, then digit preference will be expected. If digit preference is found in data that should have been machine-generated, such as electronic blood pressure readings or multichannel analyser results for biochemical tests, then this becomes good evidence that some subversion of the data has taken place. It may also be helpful to examine the pattern of digit preference by investigator in a multicentre trial and by treatment group. In one instance, so far unpublished, there was a clear difference in digit preference between the baseline measurements for several variables by treatment group, when random allocation had supposedly been performed. This constitutes evidence for some form of interference with the data.

Examining data: two measurements of the same variable

As an example, consider a trial comparing two treatments (A and B) for hypertension. A way of analysing the data is to look at the individual changes in blood pressure and compare these changes between the two groups.

The basic data consist of the values of blood pressure for each individual at randomisation (r) and at final assessment (f). A t test or confidence interval is calculated using the changes $(f-r)$, comparing groups A and B.

Statistical methods

Ordinary data checking will look for outlying values (values a long way from the mean) of blood pressure at r or f, and in the changes $(f-r)$. Fraudulent data will not usually have outlying values, rather the reverse. Outliers increase the variability of the data more than they affect the mean, so statistical significance using a t test will be reduced. When data have been manipulated by either removing or changing values that are inconvenient from the fraudster's viewpoint, or when data are completely invented, the range of data will not be extreme. The data will have the outliers removed or "shrunk" towards the mean, and some values may have small changes to increase the differences between the groups.

A sensitive test of fraud will be to find markedly reduced variability in the changes in the blood pressures. For blood pressure, and for many other variables that are measured in research, there is good knowledge of this variability. It tends not to be examined as carefully as the mean or median values that are reported. Extreme values of the mean or median will be noticed easily, but the usual reader, and even the referee and editor of a paper, will be less likely to examine the variability. For blood pressure, the between-person variability in most studies has a standard deviation of close to 10 mmHg. This variation increases with increasing mean value so that, in studies of hypertensive patients, the variability will be rather larger.

193

The within-person standard deviation varies with the length of time between the making of the measurements concerned, tending to increase as the time between measurements increases. An alternative way of looking at this is to state that the correlation between the two measurements tends to decrease the further apart they are in time. This will happen without treatment, but will also happen in the presence of treatment. Two measurements repeated within a few minutes tend to have a correlation that may be as high as 0.8, while measurements a week or so apart tend to have a correlation of about 0.6–0.7. Values several years apart tend to have lower correlations, falling to about 0.3 at 10 years. These are very approximate values, but those working in a field can obtain the relevant values from their own data that have been shown to be genuine. The within-person standard deviation then tends to be about 7 mmHg for values from one week to a few months apart, which is the typical range of time encountered in much research. The reports of studies, whether genuine or not, often tend to neglect the reporting of the variability of differences. A summary P value may be the only statistic that is given. If this P value is given exactly (rather than $P < 0.05$), then it is possible to work back to obtain an approximate original standard deviation of the differences. Hence it is possible to see if there is a hint that the data do not have the expected variability.

When changes are examined, which will always be the case when any paired statistical significance tests are done as well as when changes are compared between groups, then the variability of the changes should also be given. It is well known that comparisons in a table are made more easily by going down a column than across a row. This means that the same values in different groups should be given in columns so that comparisons may be made more easily.

The issue of variability of changes is not examined carefully enough. All too often, the baseline and final means and standard deviations are presented with just a P value for the comparison of the changes. Firstly, this makes detection of bad data more difficult; secondly, in order to plan further studies using those changes, especially when calculating sample size, the essential information is not available in the publication. This must be one of the most frequent problems encountered by the consulting statistician helping to plan sample sizes for new research.

Graphical methods

Graphical methods tend not to be used for pairs of observations although, when the pairs of points are shown joined by lines, it is possible to see when variability is too little by noting that all the lines are parallel. When the same variable is repeatedly measured, this type of graph can be used, but it is rarely done. The usual graphs do not indicate anything of the within-person variability. With modern statistical graphics it is easy to identify different centres or investigators with different plotting symbols. These can be helpful in exploratory analysis of the data rather than in graphs intended for publication.

Examining data: two or more variables at a time

Statistical methods

When data are invented to manipulate or show an effect that is not present or not present so clearly in the genuine data, then a skilled manipulator will perhaps be able to produce convincing data when viewed in one dimension. It is very much more difficult to retain the nature of real data when viewed in two dimensions. The relationship between variables tends to disappear. In a well-documented example,[9] a laboratory study on animal models of myocardial infarction involved a number of variables. The simplest example of this problem was the data relating weight of the dogs versus the weight of the left ventricle. In this example of very elaborate forgery, the range and variability of left ventricle weight was high, in fact higher than in the genuine data, with a similar range for the weights of the dogs. The correlation between these two measurements was very much weaker. The situation with infarct size versus collateral blood flow was even worse, where the variability in collateral blood flow was very much less than expected and the relationship that should have existed was absent.

This type of problem is not easy to detect by simply reading a paper, but ought to be detected by a statistician with access to the raw data and familiar with the science of the study. In some cases, a correlation matrix may be presented, and careful examination of this may show unexpected findings that raise the index of suspicion.

In the example quoted,[9] the study was being carried out in several laboratories simultaneously so that the differences between the laboratories could be studied very easily. In fact, the study itself was set up because of previous inconsistencies in the results from different laboratories.

In many situations, there are no data available from multicentre studies and considerable experience in the field may be necessary to detect the problem.

The situation with regard to several variables is an extension of that seen with two. The variables on their own tend to show reduced variability, but even when this is not so, the relationships among many variables become much weaker than they should be.

As has been noted above, the examination of the correlation matrix may also show where relationships are too weak (or, on occasions, too strong) for genuine data. This approach essentially examines the relationships between pairs of variables. True multivariate methods are able to look at the effect of many variables simultaneously. These can be of use in sophisticated data checking.

The first, well-known, multivariable method examines the "influence" of individual observations. It is of most help where data errors have been made and for ensuring that single observations do not distort the results of an analysis too much.

The basic idea is to have a single outcome variable that is the measurement of greatest importance. This is used as the response (dependent) variable in a multiple regression analysis, with a number of possible explanatory (independent) variables, including one for the treatment group if a comparative study is being analysed. The first step is to use standard methods of multiple regression. This entails obtaining as good a fit to the data as possible, which also makes biological sense. For these purposes, it may be reasonable to obtain the best fitting equation (also called a "model"), regardless of how sensible it is in biological terms. The inclusion of variables that are not thought to be medically relevant may indicate that there are problems with the data. The relationships with such variables may merit further investigation.

There are several measures of "influence" available, probably the best of them is called "Cook's distance". This is like a residual in multiple regression: the distance between an observed point and the value predicted for that point by the regression equation. It measures how far off a point is in both the X and Y directions. An ordinary residual may not be very informative, since outliers may have small residuals in that they "attract" the regression line towards them. An alternative is a "deleted" residual, which involves calculating the equation for the regression line excluding that point, and obtaining the residual from the predicted value with this regression equation. This will be very effective when a single outlying point is present in the data. An outlier can influence the regression equation in two ways. It can influence the "height" when it is in the centre of the data, but it influences the slope when it is also an outlier in at least one explanatory variable. This effect is known as "leverage", and is illustrated in Figure 14.3, where only two dimensions are shown. The usual measures of leverage effectively relate to how far points are away from the centre in the X direction. Cook's distance for the outlier in Figure 14.3b is very large because it has leverage as well as being an outlier. In Figure 14.3a it is an outlier but does not have leverage and has a smaller Cook's distance. The slope of the line in Figure 14.3b has been notably altered by a single observation. Single outliers are probably more likely to be data errors rather than invented data, but investigation of the reasons for the outlier may be important in the data analysis for genuine as well as fraudulent data. There do exist statistical tests for multiple outliers, but these are beyond the scope of this introduction but the Hadi statistic is implemented in the statistical packages Stata (College Station, Texas) and DataDesk (Ithaca, New York). Statistical mathematics will not usually be as helpful as graphics in detection of problems.

The problem with an invented data point is that it is unlikely to be an outlier in any dimension; in fact, the exact opposite is true. Invented data are likely to have values that lie close to the mean for each variable that has been measured. In one instance of invented data of which I had experience, the perpetrator used the results of an interim analysis of means of all the measured variables to generate four extra cases. For these cases, either the original data were lost, or the results did not fit the desired pattern, and the records were destroyed by the perpetrator. The means of the two "treatment"

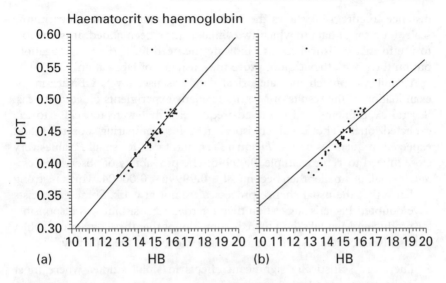

Figure 14.3 Use of Cook's distance to measure the influence of an outlying point.

groups had been provided for all haemodynamic and biochemical measurements. The perpetrator used these means as a guide so that the invented data consisted of the nearest feasible numbers close to the relevant group mean with minor changes. This meant that the data for the two individuals in each "treatment" group were similar but not absolutely identical.

These data have the effect of increasing sample size and reducing the standard deviation of every measured variable. This can have a noticeable effect on the P values – it can change from $P = 0.07$ to $P = 0.01$.

Such invented data cannot be detected by any of the usual checks. However, one method for looking for outliers can also be used to detect "inliers". It is not unusual for a value of one variable for any case to be close to the mean. It is less likely that it will be close to the mean of an entirely unrelated variable. The probability of it being close to the mean of each of a large number of variables in any individual case is then very low. The distance of a value from the mean for one variable can be expressed in units of standard deviation, a "Z score". This distance can be generalised to two dimensions when the distance from a bivariate mean (for example, diastolic blood pressure and sodium concentration each expressed as Z scores) can be calculated using Pythagoras' theorem. A measure of the distance from a multivariate mean, equivalent to the square of a Z score is called the Mahalanobis distance. The distribution of this distance should follow a *chi*-square distribution, approximately. Very large values-outliers can be detected in this way. Although not mentioned in textbooks, this can also be used to detect "inliers", looking for much smaller values of Mahalanobis

197

distance. Figure 14.4 shows the Mahalanobis distances, on a logarithmic scale, for a set of data to which two "inliers" have been added. It is possible to use formal statistical tests to indicate the need for further investigation, but on their own, they cannot prove the existence of fabrication.

A similar approach for categorical data was used by RA Fisher in his examination of the results of Mendel's genetic experiments on garden peas. Several experiments had observed frequencies that were too close to the expected ones. The usual statistical test for comparing observed and expected frequencies uses a *chi*-square test and looks for small P values very close indeed to 1, for example, 0.99996. The probability of observing a *chi-square* small or smaller then becomes $1 - 0.99996 = 0.00004$, which is strong evidence that the usual chance processes are not at work. Some geneticists have doubted Fisher's suggestion that a gardening assistant was responsible for producing Mendel's, and there is some doubt that these data are reliable, but as Fisher concludes, "There is no easy way out of the difficulty."[10]

- There are statistically significant effects in small studies where most investigators need larger ones.
- Measures of variability or standard errors are absent.

However, it is also important to realise that with any diagnostic procedure there are false positives and false negatives. If we regard a false negative as failing to recognise fraud or manipulation when it is present, then there is also the possibility of the false positive – accusing someone of fraud when it is absent. Inexperienced or ignorant investigators are particularly prone to problems with the third and fifth elements in the list above (P values without data and absence of measures of variability). This is not necessarily fraud. The guidelines on presentation of statistical evidence in Altman *et al.*[4] make it clear that these practices should be avoided. Obtaining extra evidence is the only way of reducing the rate of both these errors simultaneously. When the whiff becomes somewhat stronger, it becomes a

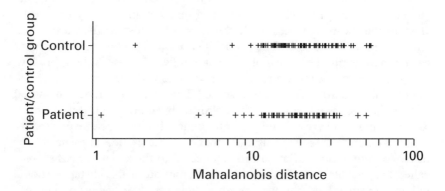

Figure 14.4 Distribution of Mahalanobis distance for a set of data to which two "inliers" have been added.

situation where the original author(s) is asked to supply the raw data. If investigators become more aware that this type of request will occur regularly, then some instances of fraud may be prevented. It must also be made clear that some of the errors found in reviewing a paper may be careless mistakes or typographic error (none of us is perfect), and some may be due to incorrect analysis through ignorance.

Graphical methods

With data in two or more dimensions, the publication of scatter plots should be encouraged whenever space permits. Modern statistical computer graphics programs can show a large number of data points in fine resolution, which are very useful for data screening. There are circumstances where such "clouds" of points can be helpful in a publication, rather than just showing a summary statistic. The mean and standard error can conceal more than they reveal.

In data checking, graphs tend to be very much more useful than numerical statistical methods, and the plotting of unusual variables against one another can show problems not found in any other way. "Unusual" implies that there is not expected to be a biological relationship of great interest between the variables. The time sequence of the data is a particularly important aspect. Altman and Royston[11] have noted the influence of time on a number of aspects of a study, although they did not mention the issue of fraud. Bailey[9] shows some dramatic pictures where the data collected by an individual extended over a time period that included both genuine and invented data, and where the time when the fraud was suspected could be seen clearly on the graph. Figure 14.5 shows that, at the site where misconduct occurred, the variability of the measurement had been very much reduced compared to other sites. When the fraudster became aware of the investigation the variability suddenly increases to the level seen at site A, where it is assumed that misconduct had not occurred.

The graphs that use the "residuals", which is the variation remaining when all the systematic and known aspects (that is the "modelled" aspects) have been removed, are especially helpful. It is in this aspect of invention that the reduced variability is seen most clearly.

Summary of steps to be taken with raw data

There are three stages of checking: firstly, routine checks; secondly, where a routine check has indicated the possibility of a problem or where some external evidence has flagged-up a particular concern and more extensive checks are required; thirdly, where there is reasonably convincing evidence of a problem of misconduct and verifying the extent of the problem or providing strong corroborative evidence towards proof of a problem is desired.

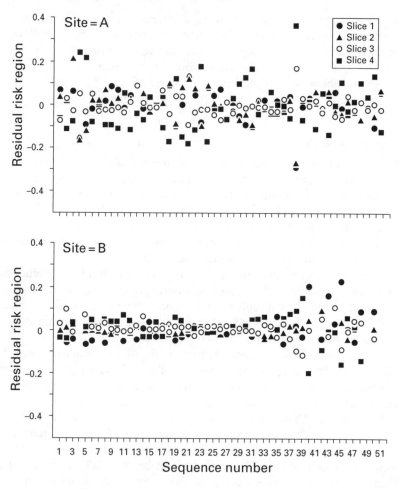

Figure 14.5 Residual risk region by sequence. Reprinted by permission of the publisher from "Detecting fabrication of data in a multicenter collaborative animal study" by KR Bailey (*Controlled Clinical Trials* 1991; **12**: 741–52). Copyright 1991 Elsevier Science Publishing Co, Inc.

Routine scanning of data

Most data are not fraudulent and it is simply not sensible, or practically possible, to scrutinise all data with a complete battery of tests for possible fraudulent data. What is required is some simple checks that go a little beyond what would be done in ordinary data checking that should be done prior to analysis of any set of data.

The first step is to examine *variability*. Comparisons may be made between centres, between treatment groups or other "interesting" groups, or with previous experience. The usual object is to look for increased variation, but it is important to also look for reduced variation. It may also

Box 14.1 Routine checking

- Variability and kurtosis
- Baseline imbalance in outcome variable
- Scatter-plot matrix by investigator/centre

be reasonable to check for baseline imbalance in the outcome variable if this is measured at baseline. Such imbalances will occur by chance on occasions, but they are particularly important in the outcome or a variable strongly correlated with the outcome. It is an indicator of misconduct when such differences are found consistently with one investigator, but are absent in data from all other investigators.

Standard statistical computer programs calculate standard deviation and usually also calculate *kurtosis*. It is a reasonable minor extra effort to check the kurtosis as well as the standard deviation.

When the obvious errors in the data have been corrected, then it is reasonable to produce a scatter plot matrix of the variables that might be expected to relate to one another. The extra work required in checking such a scatter plot, even if there are separate plots for a number of centres, will take only a few minutes. Regular use of these techniques will enable the data analyst to become familiar with the pattern shown by genuine data.

It is not difficult with computer programs to be able to obtain histograms of final digits. In some circumstances, it may be reasonable to carry out regular checking for digit preference. However, this is probably unnecessary in routine use (Box 14.1).

More extensive checking

Digit preference is clearly an area that is useful for finding definite problems. This is especially true where automatic measurements are usually made, but differences in digit preference within the same study may show that investigation is warranted.

In many trials, there are repeated observations on the same individuals. When these are summarised, the within-person variation is often not studied or, if it is, then it is examined for large values that can indicate possible data errors. Again, reduced variation is an indicator of possible misconduct. Occasionally zero variation is seen in invented data for the same person. In one instance, not published, an investigator suggested that measurement of secondary or safety variables in a trial was of no interest, so it did not matter very much if they were not measured properly. Graphical display of the individual data over time with different visits can be very helpful to show different patterns for different centres or investigators.

Cluster analysis can be employed where there is a possibility that test results have been obtained by splitting a blood sample from a single individual into two or more aliquots, and then sent for testing as if they

Box 14.2 More extensive checking

- Digit preference
- Within-individual variation – look for reduced variation
- Cluster analysis
- Mahalanobis distances

came from two or more individuals. This technique and the use of Mahalanobis distances can show observations that are too similar to one another. It is helpful if genuine duplicate samples are also available, so that it can be seen that they differ by at least as much as those that purport to come from different individuals. The use of Mahalanobis distances is not justified on a routine basis, but they are very simple to obtain with modern statistical software, and plotting them by treatment group is not arduous (Box 14.2).

Corroborative evidence

It is important to realise that unusual patterns appear in genuine data. It is easy for someone whose eyes are opened to the possibility of misconduct to see it everywhere when they have not studied a great deal of genuine data. When investigating misconduct, it is good practice to set out a protocol for the analyses, with specific null hypotheses to be tested. (A Bayesian analysis will of course also be possible and may be regarded as philosophically preferable.) This protocol will usually be able to state that a particular centre or investigator has data that differ from the others in specified ways. It is advisable for the statistician carrying out such an investigation to be supplied with data from all investigators, or as many as possible. They should also not know, if possible, the identity of the suspicious centre. They can then treat each centre in a symmetrical way and look for a centre for which there is strong evidence of divergence. Finding strong evidence, from a formal statistical analysis, is then independent evidence of misconduct. It would rarely be taken as sufficient evidence on its own, but with other evidence may prove that there really was misconduct. Fraud implies intention, and statistical analysis would not impinge on this directly.

All of the methods listed above may be used in a search for evidence, and the totality of the evidence must be used to evaluate the possible misconduct. Innocent explanations may be correct. For example, a trial found one centre with very divergent results in the treatment effect observed. It turned out on further simple investigation that this investigator was from a retirement area of the South Coast of England and the ages of all the patients were very much higher than in the other centres. There was an effect of age on the treatment and this was accepted as an explanation for divergence (Box 14.3).

Box 14.3 Corroborative evidence

- Predefine a protocol
- Use as simple methods as possible
- Consider innocent explanations

Hints for referees and editors

It is a controversial point, but as a referee, I have often wanted more data than are intended to appear in the final article. Sometimes the raw data themselves may be necessary for a proper review to take place even if, because of pressure of space, they cannot appear in the final journal article. In most cases, this request for the data has been met with alacrity, since anything that helps publication is usually of interest to the author. In a very few instances, nothing more has been heard from the author(s), which leads to definite conclusions about the quality of the work. I have had one instance where the data were supplied quickly but, where although the regression analysis produced the same results as quoted, I could not reproduce the statistical significance of the findings. Again, after raising a query, nothing more was heard by me from the authors. The problem is that obtaining the raw data, especially if not supplied in a computer-readable form, require considerable resources for carrying out full analyses to detect genuine evidence of misconduct. Carelessness alone is not fraud.

Often, no raw data are available and the scrutiniser must examine the text, tables, and graphs that are submitted. Experience and knowledge of the subject area may then mean that a whiff of suspicion arises on reading a manuscript. Various things can be done in checking the immediately available material. Some points that are indicators of problems are:

- Numbers that do not add up across a table.
- Graphs with different numbers of observations from those quoted in the text.
- P values that are quoted without the data necessary to estimate them.

References

1 Armitage P, Berry G. *Statistical methods in medical research*. 2nd edn. Oxford: Blackwell Scientific, 1987, Chapter 11.
2 Altman DG. *Practical statistics for medical research*. London: Chapman & Hall, 1991, Chapter 7.
3 Neaton JD, Bartsch GE, Broste SK, Cohen JD, Simon NM. A case of data alteration in the Multiple Risk Factor Intervention Trial (MRFIT). *Controlled Clin Trials* 1991; **12**:731–40.
4 Altman DG, Madein D, Bryant TN, Gardner MJ. *Statistics with confidence*. 2nd edn. London: BMJ Books, 2000.
5 Buyse M, George SL, Evans S, *et al.* The role of biostatistics in the prevention, detection and treatment of fraud in clinical trials. *Statist Med* 1999;**18**:3435–51.
6 Scherrer B. L'apport de la biométrie. In: *La Fraude dans les Essais Cliniques*. Paris: Medicament et Santé, STS Edition, 1991.

7 Silman A. Failure of random zero sphygmomanometer in general practice. *BMJ* 1985;**290**:1781–2.
8 Bland JM. *An introduction to medical statistics*. 3rd edn. Oxford: Oxford University Press, 2000.
9 Bailey KR. Detecting fabrication of data in a multicenter collaborative animal study. *Controlled Clin Trials* 1991;**12**:741–52.
10 Freedman D, Pisani R, Purves R, Adhikari A. *Statistics*. 2nd edn. New York: Norton, 1991.
11 Altman DG, Royston JP. The hidden effect of time. *Statist Med* 1988;**7**:629–37.

PART V
PERSONAL EXPERIENCES

15: Whistleblower

DAVID EDWARDS

In the afternoon of Friday, 23 March 1996, Dr Geoffrey Fairhurst, General Practitioner and for many years my partner, was struck off by the General Medical Council after a four-day inquiry into his misconduct of medical research. Jean Young, a research colleague based at the practice, Dr M Shah, and myself, both partners in the practice, wrote the letter to the General Medical Council which started the inquiry. Dr Fairhurst was found guilty of gross professional misconduct: specifically, he entered patients in pharmaceutical trials without their consent, altered clinical notes to allow patients to be eligible for inclusion in trials, and instructed our practice nurse to produce false ECG recordings.

Although our relief at this decision was overwhelming, there was little sense of victory, for we were tired, and feared the reaction of our colleagues and friends within the medical profession. At that time to take such action was unprecedented. Since then there have been other cases where doctors have decided to risk their careers to expose wrongdoing within the medical profession.

The practice

I joined Geoff Fairhurst in 1984 after completing my GP registrar job in Blandford, Dorset. I had trained at Southampton Medical School and worked in hospitals on the south coast culminating in my GP registrar job. The move to Merseyside was a wrench, leaving the fabulous Dorset countryside to return to the North West, where I was born and brought up. The lure was an interesting GP partnership with early parity and excellent working conditions. Dr Fairhurst was a well-known GP who had a major interest in hypertension; he lectured for a number of pharmaceutical companies and was involved in medical research.

I moved to St Helens in December 1984 with my wife, Helen. The practice was recovering from a partnership dissolution and I started work enthusiastically to rebuild it. A great bonus was the excellent out-of-hours cooperative that allowed us to pursue our interest in cycle racing; at this time Helen was a Great Britain International Rider and had just ridden the 1984 Tour de France Feminin. The major surprise was the low practice profit given the good list size. In retrospect, I feel that was because

Dr Fairhurst was making a substantial part of his income from pharmaceutical trials, so income from the practice was less important to him. I was not interested in medical research at this time and became involved in the NHS work and practice administration. As we had no practice manager, I gave myself a crash course in accounting, practice administration, and wages. Dr Fairhurst was involved in local medical politics, serving on the local medical committee and local ethics committee and lecturing frequently on hypertension and his own research. This would entail frequent short trips abroad, some of them covered by locums, some not, which was the only source of irritation for me at the time.

Over the first few years of partnership it was apparent that all trial work was carried out during surgery time. This would mean that an average surgery for Dr Fairhurst might contain as many as four trial patients. Knowing little about the difficulties of pharmaceutical trials, I assumed that this practice was normal. Later, when I became acquainted with the nature of this type of work, I marvelled at his ability to manage drug accountability, arrange investigations, and discuss consent in the limited time available in a regular surgery.

Uncertainties

It is impossible to be precise when I first started to worry about the way Dr Fairhurst's research work was conducted. During the early 1990s he was employing a research assistant, Debbie, to help with the day-to-day workload while he was recruiting patients for a number of cardiovascular studies running concurrently.

Inevitably during his holidays or trips abroad lecturing, his patients would encounter problems with their trial medication. One particular incident involved a trial patient whose liver function tests were abnormal. Debbie brought these to my attention, as she was worried about the significance of the results. I arranged to see the patient to discuss this and was shocked to discover that he was completely unaware that he was taking study medication. Another incident involved a patient whom I visited at home; she needed urgent admission to hospital and, while listing her medication in the admission letter, I came across clearly labelled study drugs. She too was completely unaware that she was in a pharmaceutical trial. These incidents were separated by about 18 months and were not recorded by me at the time. I tried to dismiss their significance and doubted the patient's memory or put it down to the stress of the situation and their illness. It was some time before I began to suspect my partner of entering patients into studies without their consent. It was very difficult to accept that a doctor so well respected by his colleagues could behave in such a way.

Most of Dr Fairhurst's patients were completely in awe of him. He was a large man with a charming manner and a great repertoire of jokes. Many patients said that they often forgot why they had come to see him, as he was such a conversationalist and raconteur. There are a great many patients with hypertension in any general practice and most of them appreciate special attention. This was exactly what they got while they were entered in a study: regular blood tests, electrocardiographs, and detailed enquiry into their well-being. In consequence, most patients were grateful for the special treatment they received and seemed unconcerned that they were testing new medication, mostly angiotensin-converting enzyme inhibitors and angiotensin-II receptor antagonists.

Consent to be in these studies did not seem to worry the patients on the rare occasions when I discussed this with them. They thought Dr Fairhurst a marvellous man and eminent doctor who could do no wrong in their eyes. My dilemma was complete; a well-respected and connected colleague, loved by his patients, whom I suspected was behaving unethically and dangerously. At that time complaints about doctors' conduct were rare and were usually brought to the attention of the General Medical Council by aggrieved patients. I had never heard of a doctor blowing the whistle on a colleague.

I knew that Dr Fairhurst had had previous partners, some of whom had left after bitter arguments with him. Although he was generally good natured, when confronted with criticism of his behaviour or medical management he could become very belligerent and stubborn. If he could not get his own way on these occasions he would refer to his large personal list size and popularity. He would clearly state that he was prepared to dissolve the partnership and retain all his patients, effectively leaving his colleagues without a future. We had already lost a third partner, who had been threatened in this way following her complaint about his personal conduct.

I had a young family, mortgage, and a half share of large practice loans, so he had a very effective bargaining tool and one I had no answer to. Leaving the practice would have meant borrowing to repay the loans and finding another partnership. An additional worry was that any reference from him would probably have been of little help in finding another job. There was little I could do at that time but continue to work with him and to note any trial irregularities when they occurred.

Around this time I started to participate in a few pharmaceutical trials myself, most of them studying patients with asthma. I was amazed at the amount of time they took up. Dedicated sessions were necessary to provide the time for informed consent and the extensive examination and investigation. The drug reconciliation was often a logistic nightmare and meticulous care had to be taken. With this personal experience of the difficulties involved in this type of medical work, my suspicions grew that Dr Fairhurst simply could not be working to the protocols because of the limited time he allocated. I became very unhappy with my situation within the practice and increasingly concerned for the well-being of patients entered in his studies. I believed that Dr Fairhurst was so well respected by colleagues and patients that my concerns would not be listened to locally. I was trapped.

Crisis

In the winter of 1993 events took a turn that focused my attention on the problem and made me explore my own feelings further when a new partner and a medical researcher joined the practice.

Dr Min Shah had just finished vocational training and this was her first partnership. I found her extremely likeable and honest and soon developed a good working relationship with her. Jean Young had worked for ICI, and latterly Zeneca, for many years in its research department. She was a highly qualified nurse and had met Dr Fairhurst many years ago when he was working in a Liverpool hospital. She had decided to set up her own business coordinating pharmaceutical trials. Geoff had suggested that she rented a room in our surgery and work from the practice, recruiting patients from our list. She was a forthright and honest woman and I had no problems in agreeing to this proposal. Before long Jean came to me with her own concerns regarding Dr Fairhurst's conduct in his trials. She was concerned regarding lack of informed consent and poor drug accountability. She had discovered this while assisting Dr Fairhurst with his work while he was on holiday.

Dr Shah soon had her own suspicions that Geoff's research work was not being conducted ethically. She had quickly attracted a number of patients who were upset by the frequency of investigations requested by Dr Fairhurst. It was apparent to her that these were patients with hypertension who appeared to be taking or had taken study medication.

To her great consternation it was also clear that many were unaware that they were enrolled in pharmaceutical trials. Crucially Dr Shah discovered a signed consent form in a patient's notes relating to a study. When this consent was shown to the patient, she declared the signature was not hers. This was to become part of the evidence presented to the General Medical Council.

At this time I became further involved when an elderly patient died of digoxin toxicity. It was clear that this was due to her having two medicine bottles of digoxin at home and taking them simultaneously. She was also enrolled in a study, a fact I confirmed with the sponsoring pharmaceutical company. I was horrified to find that Dr Fairhurst had altered, in his handwriting, hospital consultants' letters and entries in her medical records made by myself. The effect of these alterations was to change the medical record to make the patient eligible for inclusion into his study. I knew that the alterations had no basis in fact as I had been seeing her regularly until a few months previously. The study involved two medicines that were available on prescription. To complete the deception and to avoid having to get patient consent or arouse suspicion, the study medicine packs were being discarded and NHS prescriptions issued for their equivalents.

My conclusion was that during the substitution of prescription for study medicine the extra digoxin had been supplied in error. I discussed these developments with Dr Shah and Mrs Young and immediately contacted my medical defence organisation and the medical director of the pharmaceutical company involved.

Advice from the defence organisation was vague and unhelpful, apart from the simple fact that we had a duty to report our concerns to a responsible body, probably the General Medical Council. The medical director of the drug company was quite clear that he could not believe my story and that Dr Fairhurst was well respected in this area of research and personally known to him. He then contacted Dr Fairhurst and reported the details of our conversation to him. We needed help and we needed it fast so I contacted the General Medical Council for guidance. They sent me information, intended for patients, outlining the complaints procedures. I now knew that a complaint brought some years previously to the local medical committee about Dr Fairhurst's conduct of pharmaceutical studies had not been taken further and, to complicate matters, Dr Fairhurst sat on the local ethical committee. We feared the old boy network and did not wish to present the matter locally; as a consequence we were floundering and did not know where to turn.

I approached Dr Fairhurst with my concerns regarding his research work. As expected, he denied that there were any problems and insisted that all his work was being done ethically. He concluded the meeting with the expected suggestion that he would dissolve our partnership and take the majority of the patients with him. A friend in the pharmaceutical industry suggested that we contact the Association of the British Pharmaceutical Industry. This organisation, and in particular its then medical director, Dr Frank Wells, was to be a great source of help and support.

Action

In mid-December 1994 we approached Dr Wells and met to discuss our problem. He clarified our position confirming that we had a professional duty to report our concerns to the General Medical Council. In the following three months from December 1994 to February 1995 we discovered further evidence in the medical records of patients, including forged consent forms and appointment diaries clarifying how electrocardiographs (ECGs) were to be produced with fictitious dates. Up to three electrocardiograms were recorded from a patient consecutively. The date recorded by the machine on the tracing was changed between each ECG so that it appeared as if the traces had been recorded on different dates and times over a three-month period. Our practice nurse had been asked to do this on a regular basis by Dr Fairhurst. He could thus complete trial data quickly with the minimum of effort. It is a testimony to his charm and charisma that our nurse had been complying for some time with these requests. We were uneasy about our role at this time as we were almost acting as investigators; however, we knew that, to succeed, our case would have to be strong and supported by documentary evidence. All of the patients involved were shocked at the discovery of the falsified consent

211

forms but all confirmed in writing that the signatures on the forms were not theirs.

Once completed, the document ran to many pages and was posted to the General Medical Council in February 1995. I felt as if the long fuse to a bomb had been lit. We waited many weeks for a reply from the General Medical Council. When it finally arrived it was a postcard explaining that the matter was receiving their attention. You can imagine our irritation, as there was nothing there to allay our fears and everyday work became almost unbearable because of the anxiety.

To clarify our position we contacted the British Medical Association (BMA) and the local industrial relations officer was extremely helpful. He accompanied us when we met the health authority to inform them of our action. The chief executive and medical director were obviously shocked but explained that they were unable to take any action or help us, and would await the General Medical Council's decision.

In July 1995 Geoff Fairhurst wrote to Dr Shah and myself to inform us he was ending his partnership with us. He would become single-handed, taking his 3500 patients, and share the jointly owned surgery with me. However, he gave me notice to quit our branch surgery, where we had around 2500 patients. Dr Shah decided to leave the practice and found another partnership locally. I had just a month to arrange alternative accommodation for my 1000 patients at the branch surgery and make arrangements for 2400 patients in total. With a friend I purchased a house nearby and obtained planning permission to convert it into a surgery. There would not be enough time to convert the premises and Dr Fairhurst would not contemplate an extension to the deadline. Fortunately a local general practitioner, Khalid Laghari, contacted me, offering to share his premises with me. These were only a few hundred yards away and the move was completed without problem or inconvenience to anyone. During that period I was very concerned that I would lose many of my patients and would not have a viable practice. I continue to work from Khalid's surgery and believe that his generous action ensured the viability of my practice.

The next year was a very stressful time both at work and at home. At times it was difficult to concentrate or find enjoyment in anything. My wife, Helen, had been involved since my first suspicions and had been supportive and encouraging from the start, but the state of affairs placed a great strain on our relationship. We discussed each twist and turn and, when Dr Fairhurst dissolved the partnership, Helen chose to become my practice manager. She had a degree in history and politics and brought many office skills to the practice and helped to manage change through a very difficult period for the staff. From my selfish point of view it was reassuring to have someone I could trust completely to manage the practice, and for Helen there was the advantage of viewing the problems at first hand. Even so those three years were a terrible torment for us both. I was worried about the effect the action might have on my career, so for insurance we applied for immigration documents for Australia.

During the period between the dissolution of the partnership in July 1995 and the General Medical Council hearing in March 1996, Dr Fairhurst was informed by them of the details of our complaints against him. I continued to work in the same building and our respective staff had to share the office and equipment. To look back, it is amazing that we could continue working normally during this period. All my staff are still working with me and their support and loyalty was invaluable. The health authority was aware of the difficulties of the situation and assisted where possible, but this was confined to chairing meetings and arbitrating between the two practices: for all practical purposes, we were on our own during this time, with no support locally. Dr Fairhurst continued to practise and sit on the local medical and ethics committees and lobbied for his cause, spreading misinformation to patients and colleagues in the area. As the date of the hearing approached, the tension built both at home and within the practice. There were no second thoughts now and even the patients involved were committed to their day under the spotlight.

The Hearing

The Professional Conduct Committee held the inquiry between the 21st and 24th of March 1996 at the General Medical Council. My imagination had worked overtime in the preceding months and the venue and the cast did not disappoint me. The General Medical Council has imposing premises, and the room in which the hearing took place was very similar to a courtroom. The committee and chairman sat at the front of the chamber with the opposing lawyers on either side. Dr Fairhurst sat with his counsel throughout and a public gallery containing the press and friends overlooked the whole spectacle. Witnesses were not allowed to observe from the gallery until they had given their evidence and been cross-examined. Until our turns came, all witnesses were seated in a small adjoining chamber, where we read and tried to pass the time. Everyone was tense and conversation was difficult.

I recollect that I gave evidence and was cross-examined for about three hours – at least it seemed that long to me. Dr Fairhurst's defence was intent on discrediting my character and proving that the complaint against him was malicious. During the questioning I was concentrating on answering the questions precisely and honestly and did not find it distressing. However, others felt that it had been vitriolic and at times rather too personal. The hearing lasted a total of three and a half days and was an emotional rollercoaster as the case unfolded.

The most impressive witnesses were the patients who had been involved; their testimony was very powerful and moving, and all stated clearly that they had never consented verbally or in writing to be entered in any research studies. Their evidence was supported by consent forms containing false signatures and a great deal of evidence obtained by the General Medical Council from the pharmaceutical companies involved.

The official investigation had uncovered many irregularities in Dr Fairhurst's running of trials and we felt thoroughly vindicated.

The most disturbing event for me was the character reference from the Chairman of St Helens and Knowsley Local Medical Committee, Dr Colin Ford, who, after Dr Fairhurst was found guilty, stated that the committee maintained its confidence in Dr Fairhurst and wished him to remain a member of the committee and to represent them on the ethical committee dealing in matters such as drug trials. I took this as a sign of local medical opinion and felt hugely let down by my colleagues.

On the Friday afternoon the committee found Dr Fairhurst guilty of serious professional misconduct and directed that his name be removed from the register. Dr Shah, Jean Young, and I walked out of the General Medical Council together, braving the TV and radio reporters before quickly disappearing into the busy London streets.

Aftermath

It was work as usual on the Monday and, apart from some disparaging graffiti painted on the surgery front door and kind words of support from some bold patients, the day passed quietly. Our health authority showed its sensitivity by employing Dr Fairhurst's daughter to work in the office at the shared surgery. I am still amazed by this action to this day. The atmosphere was very difficult during those first few weeks until she returned to college.

There were a number of patients, friends, and colleagues of Dr Fairhurst who believed that a terrible error had been made and that he was innocent. Unfortunately the discredited doctor encouraged these people and a support group was started. They tried to make life difficult for me for the next eighteen months with spurious and unfounded allegations, holding local fund raising meetings to finance their cause. The group gradually lost momentum when Dr Fairhurst failed to appeal against the General Medical Council decision, his patients were reassigned to another practice, and the promised exposure of my own wrongdoing failed to materialise. Their action did upset and disturb my family and interfered with my professional life, which I believe was what they intended. What was of greater concern was the future of our jointly owned surgery and how the practice financial affairs would be resolved. This took a further four years and many thousands of pounds in solicitors' fees to resolve.

Geoff Fairhurst and I had joint debts relating to the surgery of around £60 000 in addition to the mortgage. The bank had great difficulty in contacting Dr Fairhurst to discuss repayment of his half of the loans. After two years of constant telephone calls and meetings with the bank, it became obvious that it was prepared, as a last resort, to pursue me for the total amount. It was unable to persuade Geoff Fairhurst to meet and discuss the situation and we became very anxious about our finances. In addition, until this was resolved we were unable to make any investment in the practice or plan for our future. Eventually the bank, after much discussion, persuasion, and help from the medical establishment, decided to divide the debt in half and I repaid my share. The British Medical Association were supportive and helpful during this period of difficulty and their advice was invaluable.

The problem of the surgery premises took a little longer to resolve, and for four years we were unable to use some of the rooms on the insistence of Dr Fairhurst's solicitors. These restrictions precluded my advertising for a partner so I remained single-handed for this period.

Eventually an agreement was struck whereby I bought Dr Fairhurst's share in the surgery and I now wholly own the surgery. The anxiety and stress of the financial complications were unforeseen and were as great as the initial action itself. It was clear throughout this period that, although doctors have a duty to protect patients, there is no mechanism to protect the whistleblowing doctor from the financial repercussions of his or her action. The health authority has no mandate to help in this unusual situation, and I could fully understand a doctor being reluctant to act for fear of financial hardship. The anachronistic partnership laws do not help in these difficult circumstances and, without goodwill, disputes could last interminably.

We have now become a second wave PMS pilot and two doctors and a nurse clinician have joined the team. I am teaching students from Liverpool Medical School one day a week and my enthusiasm for medicine has never been greater.

At the time our action was unprecedented. It succeeded because we were united and committed to exposing the truth. I would not have been able to bring this case to the General Medical Council without the commitment and determination of Dr Min Shah and Jean Young. I know that there are other doctors working in similar situations who are unable for many good reasons to take any action. I hope that recent cases will have raised awareness and alerted professional bodies to the difficulties faced by whistleblowers so that our own experiences are not repeated.

16: Research fraud/ misconduct: a glance at the human side

PETER JAY

In the UK the integrity of the scientific database would seem to have been of little interest to criminal law, health ministers and successive governments, professional bodies and the universities, or indeed to the average man in the street. The one sector which has shown some interest and which has provided support for maintaining that integrity is the pharmaceutical industry. However, to skew the scientific database is an affront to science, scientists, sponsors of research, and those doctors – fortunately the vast majority – whose standards remain high. The dishonesty of a small minority of doctors who cheat, forge and fabricate in the conduct of clinical trials, creates havoc and pain for far more innocent people than the average man would realise. The degree of that havoc and pain should not be underestimated and there is a clear message from the patients who are exploited that their safety must be given priority.

The purpose of this chapter is therefore to show what can be done, informally, to put into place an effective mechanism for the prevention, detection, investigation, and prosecution of those persons – mainly doctors – who commit biomedical research misconduct or fraud, where no formal arrangements exist. The absence of official recognition to have in place a formal pathway for the investigation of alleged research misconduct has led to the establishment of a private independent agency, supported by the pharmaceutical industry, which fulfils this role. MedicoLegal Investigations Limited (MLI), the agency in question, could be compared to an unwanted pregnancy. For years in the UK there have been unanswered representations for an official body to handle suspected research misconduct. Whilst those who mattered agreed it was essential, there was no delivery. Although MLI was not what had been asked for, they have generally been accepted as the (perhaps provisional) answer. As an investigator with the solicitors of the British doctors' disciplinary body, the General Medical Council (GMC) and therefore having extensive experience of handling misconduct in all forms, it was clear that the cases which surfaced represented only a proportion of the total number likely to be committing fraud. They also featured dishonest doctors who had been up to no good for so long, that their total disregard for the possibility of detection indicated arrogance in the extreme. Their misdeeds were blatantly obvious. This in itself posed a worrying question: "Just how many fraudsters are avoiding detection?" There was a need for something to be done. MLI has now been in operation for over five years, formed as an amalgam of two individuals – one a detective, the other a doctor – who had, sequentially, been involved in the preparation of a number of cases of indisputable research fraud for disciplinary hearings in front of the General Medical Council, all of them found guilty of serious professional misconduct.

The mentality of the fraudster is interesting in itself. The avoidance of detection is a game; much personal satisfaction is derived from the power to deceive, whilst the luck of being caught, then let off free, is sheer encouragement to be fraudulent again. The "skill" is then enhanced by lessons learned and it becomes far harder to detect next time. A dishonest individual will regard the verbal warning as a demonstration of weakness rather than kindness or fairness.

The investigation of research misconduct by MLI brings them into frequent contact with patients. It is important then to explain the process for making contact and the manner in which patients who may (or may not) have been exploited are handled.

Pharmaceutical company monitors do not interview patients neither do they see documents that could lead to the identification of patients. They are in receipt of initials and dates of birth of those participating in studies but have to rely very heavily upon the integrity of the doctor employed as investigator at whatever site, hospital or general practice. The monitoring process requires access to source data as well as anonymised records created by the doctor, plus consent forms and patient diary cards. Once suspicions are raised and a MLI investigation is requested, the process follows a well-trodden path.

All information originating from the company is double-checked and as much corroboration as possible is gathered. Only when there are very good reasons to believe that patient safety may be in jeopardy, or exploitation is probable, are efforts made to make contact with patients. This is done through health authorities who maintain computer records of patients listed with general practitioners, or NHS Trusts if hospital-based research is under scrutiny. Carefully worded letters are sent to patients informing them that some research in which they may (or may not) have taken part is "being reviewed". The letters do not cause alarm but they do produce a 70% response rate and are sent by the relevant authority without MLI being informed of patient identities. Patients are asked to respond by completing a tear-off slip with their names, addresses, and telephone numbers agreeing to be seen informally at their homes or any other convenient location. Interviews are conducted sensitively and with great care. Although a frequent response is limited to three words – "Study?

217

What study?" – it is always possible that the doctor under investigation is guilty of nothing more than sloppy work. This is why no mention is made of "fraud" or "misconduct" until evidence to support such reference is available.

No information is passed to MLI regarding the identities of the patients; the health authority simply addresses the envelopes containing the letters. Data Protection legislation created an initial hurdle in that the use of data held on record by organisations has to be recorded in registration applications to the Data Protection Registrar (DPR), at the time of registration. The forwarding of letters to patients in such circumstances as these was not covered. However, correspondence between MLI and the DPR resulted in the acceptance of special circumstances. The latter used as a test for justification the anticipated wishes of patients, should someone suitably qualified suspect their exploitation. It was quite ridiculous to believe that the law could protect a dishonest practitioner from exposure and fail to protect patients whose safety might be in jeopardy.

Written statements are taken from patients if evidence of misconduct emerges. They are told that it might be necessary to attend a hearing in London. Anger arising from exploitation, worries about future healthcare and notions of revenge through litigation are addressed, as far as possible, at the time. No patient is ever given bad news and then left alone to ponder the implications.

Once completed, the case papers are passed to the sponsoring company for assessment by their lawyers before being sent to the General Medical Council. If no evidence emerges from such an investigation the matter stops there. No one sets out to "make a case" regardless, and no doctor should fear the chance of a mistake leading to his appearance at the General Medical Council. These investigations focus upon areas of dishonesty or recklessness so serious that misconduct has, in all probability, occurred.

The monitoring process is by no means the only mechanism for finding suspicion. Whistleblowers play a major role and partners in general practice or nurses are the most common sources of information. Chairmen of Local Research Ethics Committees (LRECs) have been known to receive complaints from patients direct; several NHS Trusts have reacted positively to their own concerns and a number of health authorities have reported incidents to MLI that led to investigations.

Once misconduct is clearly established at a given site, the Chairman of the LREC is notified and asked to supply a list of studies approved in the previous five years for that particular "investigator". The medical directors of all sponsoring pharmaceutical companies are then notified. They have three main choices. They may wish to take no action (usually if the development of a medication under trial has been abandoned for commercial reasons or lack of efficacy). They can arrange a "for-cause" audit or commission a full investigation by MLI. So devious are some of the deceptions perpetrated, that companies often come back to MLI stating that they are satisfied, beyond all doubt, with the integrity of the data in their particular study. However, in the light of our experience, they will usually still commission a full investigation and, in two recent cases, all patients shown as participating in apparently "squeaky clean" studies posed the same question when interviewed, "Study, what study?". The companies were horrified to find that they had been deceived.

The obtaining of public domain information from LRECs is motivated by concerns about patient safety and product licence applications. To read in the press of a doctor being struck off the Medical Register and realising that he was one of the main investigators in a study, the database for which was closed the day before, is very worrying indeed for a pharmaceutical company.

Once an investigator has been shown beyond all reasonable shadow of doubt to have submitted fraudulent data to a pharmaceutical company or contract house, it is essential in the interests of the public, the profession, and the industry that the doctor should be dealt with in a forthright manner, either by appropriate disciplinary process or by prosecution. In the UK referral to the General Medical Council is considered appropriate, for consideration by the Professional Conduct Committee.

An example of the cases in which MLI has been fully involved involves Dr Geoffrey Fairhurst, who, in the mid-1990s was in partnership with a much younger doctor, Dr David Edwards, whose own investigations worried him enormously, leading him to seek the help of Dr Frank Wells. Together they managed to assemble a case sufficient to trigger Preliminary Proceedings at the General Medical Council. Examples of other cases appear in Chapter 5 by Wells and the viewpoint of the whistleblower in the Fairhurst case features in Chapter 15 by Edwards.

Dr Fairhurst had exploited several of his older patients by involving them in clinical trials without their knowledge and taking samples of their blood or ECG tracings which he then used ostensibly as if from other patients. When Fairhurst faced the Professional Conduct Committee of the General Medical Council, he was found guilty of serious professional misconduct and the Committee made some important comments that exemplify the importance given to this type of case and that are therefore worth setting out in full:

Dr Fairhurst, trust lies at the heart of the practice of medicine. Patients must be able to trust doctors with their lives and well being. That trust must not be abused. Medical research is fundamental to the advance of medical practice and must always be conducted with scrupulous honesty and integrity. Where doctors intend to involve patients in clinical trials, it is essential they first give those patients a proper explanation. Patients have the right to know what is involved, and to understand the implications for them, before they are invited to take part. No such trial should ever be carried out without the consent of the patient. The trust of the patients is maintained through such understanding and consent.

The facts proved against you in the charge demonstrate that you have repeatedly behaved dishonestly and have betrayed the trust placed in you by your patients, in particular by involving them in pharmaceutical trials without their knowledge or consent. You have also abused the trust of your medical colleagues and those with whom you were collaborating in pharmaceutical trials. In doing so, you have undermined the reputation of the medical profession, and damaged the confidence of the public in the integrity of scientific research. Your behaviour has not only been dishonourable in itself, but has also placed the welfare of patients at risk.

In your case the Committee's concern is the greater because of the position you have held as a member of a Local Research Ethics Committee. The Committee have judged you to have been guilty of serious professional misconduct in relation to the facts proved against you in the charge, and have directed the Registrar to erase your name from the Register. The effect of the foregoing direction is that unless you exercise your right of appeal, your name will be erased from the Register 28 days from today.

Finally, the Committee wish me to add the following statement. All doctors are reminded of their duty to take action where they have good reason, as in this case, to believe that a colleague may be acting contrary to the standards of practice set out in the Council's guidance. Only in this way can the Council uphold the integrity of the profession.

The case of Dr Geoffrey Fairhurst highlighted a number of issues. The Committee's comments were more lengthy than usual and sent out a very clear message to the medical profession that it would not tolerate behaviour of that kind. It also recognised the plight of the whistleblower and emphasised the responsibilities of individual doctors who suspected wrongdoing. Fairhurst had been dishonest for a long time – the evidence clearly demonstrated that fact – but he was allowed to continue with the exploitation of patients and skewing the scientific database because no one stopped him. There used never to be a mechanism in place to deal with such matters and dishonest doctors were able to learn from their mistakes and take precautions to ensure that detection was harder in the future.

Curiously, in spite of all the evidence and publicity, and with representatives of a group of patients in support of Fairhurst present at the hearing, there was still belief in St Helens (near Liverpool) that he was the victim. There were meetings and collections for funds to fight his appeal. No appeal materialised.

Much criticism has been levelled against the establishment in the UK that no action has yet been taken to set up an official body to which all cases of research misconduct could be referred without prejudice and without delay for advice and, if necessary, investigation. Meanwhile, however, the informal investigatory mechanism described in this chapter has provided a service, which has enabled successful action to be taken against a significant number of fraudsters, using the formal disciplinary mechanism provided by the General Medical Council.

There are alternative legal options open to complainants within the UK and, obviously, in other countries. As far as the UK is concerned, in clinical research cases where there is *prima facie* evidence of exploitation and/or fabrication, there is a priority for considering whether or not the practitioner in question should continue to practise as a doctor. For that reason the chosen route is to the General Medical Council. However, one might argue that the potential for imprisonment in such serious matters is a live consideration when the merits of criminal proceedings are being pondered.

The problem with that lies with the degree of criminal responsibility. Forgery of documents may be difficult to prove, as handwriting evidence, although much stronger now, is easy to challenge. The obtaining (or attempting to obtain) money by deception from a pharmaceutical company for bogus research might be serious enough to justify a fine for a first offender but unlikely to merit imprisonment. The full act of obtaining by deception carries a maximum 10 years' imprisonment, but this is for persistent offenders. A first offender is unlikely to receive a stiff punishment, particularly as any lawyer will make it clear to the trial judge that the doctor will still have to face his own professional body once found guilty of a criminal offence. Leniency should therefore be anticipated. A criminal trial can take two years to materialise during which time a doctor may continue to practise.

Criminal proceedings will inevitably create difficulties for the legal process. Convincing a jury of guilt in cases where a seemingly charming doctor protests his innocence would be difficult in the extreme, especially if they do not understand the intricacies of clinical trials. The real fraudster has to be an accomplished actor otherwise he could not perpetrate deceptions. For these reasons, the UK's preferred route for bringing the medical perpetrator of clinical research fraud to justice is via the body which regulates the medical profession – the General Medical Council.

There is, however, no reason to prevent a complainant pharmaceutical company seeking to recover its financial losses, either in cases where a doctor has been found guilty of serious professional misconduct or as an alternative to GMC proceedings. It must be remembered that in cases where a doctor has obtained a few thousand pounds dishonestly, his actions overall may have been responsible for losses totalling hundreds of thousands of pounds. With that in mind it will happen, one day, that a complainant pharmaceutical company will seek full compensation under civil law.

Temptation to cut corners is always present in commerce. Conflicts of interest between profits, speed of product development, and patient safety are ever-present. Pharmaceutical companies carry a huge weight of responsibility to ensure that research and development have patient safety and scientific integrity as priorities over commercial interests. Some examples of irresponsibility witnessed by MLI have indicated a naïve rather than reckless approach. For example, as a cost-saving exercise, a lone auditor may be sent to investigate concerns at a particular site. If dishonesty is suspected there must be two auditors – lack of corroboration may later weaken any proceedings and, in any event, the individual employee needs to be protected against a malicious response to his/her reports of malpractice.

One resounding message must be emphasised: whether we like it or not, fraud happens. When it happens in the clinical research context, patients are exploited, sponsoring companies or institutions are abused, and scientific integrity is compromised. It is in the interests of society that these are minimised and MLI will continue to strive to meet this objective.

PART VI
THE ROLE OF THE EDITOR

17: Fraud and misconduct in medical research: prevention

LESLEY H REES

Prevention cannot be discussed without first attempting to identify the causes. As will become apparent, because of the lack of real evidence and hard data, this will remain a largely speculative exercise. Is fraud and misconduct in medical research a new phenomenon or was it ever thus? Was the culture such that it was deemed inimical to even question the integrity of one's scientific colleagues in the past? On the other hand, is this merely a reflection of the current state of the mores of society at the present time? A random glance at the current newspapers and periodicals shows the crime rate in the UK to be the highest in the developed world apart from Australia (*Economist* 3 March 2001). In the same issue of this periodical Sotheby's former chief executive was found guilty of collusion with Christies with regard to sales of art works. Finally, in *The Times* (3 March 2001) the Automobile Association admitted plagiarising Ordnance Survey (OS) original maps and paid the OS £20 million in an out of court settlement.

It was the high profile Darsee fraud, which came to light exactly 30 years ago, that sowed the seeds of the idea that there might be a significant amount of fraud and misconduct in scientific biomedical research (see Chapters 3 and 4). Prior to that time this would have been unthinkable. However, since then, the publicity accorded several other celebrated examples has led to a greater emphasis on the detection of misconduct as well as attempts to determine its prevalence and to understand and diagnose the motivation lying behind such deceptions. It is generally believed, without much evidence, that this greater understanding should enable more effective prevention.

The previous editions of this book did not have a chapter entitled "Prevention", although many of the issues were embedded in the other contributions, in particular that of Povl Riis when he discussed the Danish experience.[1,2] Instead, most of the literature has focused on the methodology employed in detecting and dealing with it, rather than the ways of preventing it. Perhaps, there was no chapter in the previous editions solely devoted to prevention because the evidence base of what can be done to prevent research misconduct is mainly absent. Of course this does not mean that we should not try; indeed we have to, because the consequences of research misconduct have profound implications for us all: the public, our patients, and the whole scientific community.

The spectrum of scientific misconduct, defined by the Commission established by the Danish Medical Research Council in 1991, is comprehensive, and they prefer the term "scientific dishonesty" to cover a wide spectrum of offences rather than "fraud or misconduct". This is useful when we consider prevention, because it is my personal belief that the establishment of a culture that prevents the more "minor" dishonesties is likely to prevent major fraud, the latter having huge consequences for society at large. The Consensus Statement of the Royal College of Physicians of Edinburgh, published in January 2000,[3] defined research misconduct as "behaviour by a researcher, intentional or not, that falls short of good ethical and scientific standards". It also stated that no definition can or should attempt to be exhaustive and that it should allow for change. Most of the consensus statement focused on the promotion of good research in the belief that it is only within a culture of best research practices that prevention will occur.

The research culture

In 1989 a report from the Institute of Medicine in the USA[4] highlighted the importance of training new scientists in research standards and ethics. Indeed, in the USA as elsewhere, training is now required for, amongst others, those enrolling in research training and in receipt of grants from the National Institutes of Health (NIH) or the Alcohol, Drug Abuse, and Mental Health Administration (ADAMHA). In the UK, the Medical Research Council (MRC) requires that the code of Good Research Practice (GRP) is adhered to.[5,6] Ten years ago, a survey of more than 2000 biomedical trainees (clinicians and basic scientists, medical students, graduates, and postdoctoral fellows) at the University of California in San Diego found that 23% had no training in research ethics, 36% had observed some kind of scientific misconduct and 15% would be willing to select, omit, or fabricate data to win a grant or publish a paper.[7]

Even more alarming was a report that, in a survey of 1000 students in UK universities by Newstead and colleagues in 1994, 12% admitted copying from a neighbour during an examination and 8% stated that they had taken crib sheets into the examination hall (*Independent*, 26 March 1994).

In the UK in 1998, a paper in the Association of Medical Schools in Europe Newsletter (AMSE) drew attention to the extensive repercussions and fall-out from research misconduct, drawing extensively on the USA experience, which is discussed by others in this book. The University of Chicago responded by developing a two-year "scientific integrity" programme and concluded that, when a new researcher joins an institution (university, medical school, research institute, or hospital), research misconduct will not be tolerated.[8] This bottom-up approach is really the only practical way of creating the right culture, which must start with undergraduate education (both medical and scientific) and extend within the framework of lifelong learning and continuing educational and professional development. In order to achieve this, however, systems must be in place to ensure formal training of those responsible for research supervision and the establishment of written codes of best practice. In the case of the fraudulent papers published by Pearce and colleagues (1995) (see Chapter 4), no such procedures were in place, and some of the younger investigators were the hapless victims of the gross research misconduct.[9] In the case of Davies in 1999 (see Chapter 4), younger colleagues participating in the research were subjected to threats and abuse for failing to comply with the demands of the senior investigator. It is to their credit that they blew the whistle, which initiated the investigations resulting in Davies being erased from the Medical Register by the GMC.

Every institution engaged in research must have a manual of good practice that clearly states the responsibilities of both the research worker and the supervisor. It should be made clear that there must be regular discussions between the two about the data and the progress of the research. Access to raw data must be readily available and subject to external review when appropriate. It must also be explicit that the raw data do not belong to the individual researcher or supervisor but to the institution itself.[10] This requires meticulous recording and accessibility of research data, and these records cannot "travel" (except in duplicated form) with the research worker or supervisor; the raw data must also be available for at least ten years after publication. In the main, the pharmaceutical industry, for obvious reasons, has long had these good practices in place, which probably accounts for the fact that most proven examples of research misconduct arise from within the industry, attesting and providing "evidence" that their procedures expose fraud more effectively than in other domains of the scientific community. In this regard external audit by examiners who demand to see the raw data should be welcomed, and the assistance of trained statisticians employed. If this had been the case, it is arguable that one of the Pearce papers might not have been published, although in truth uncertainty about this still exists.[9] As discussed in Chapter 18, editors and their teams have an important role to play.

Whilst it may be relatively easy for the right research culture to be established in an individual organisation, multicentred trials and collaborations carry their own difficulties, especially when conducted across international boundaries and differing cultural backdrops. At the outset, transparency must be the name of the game, and issues of authorship clearly spelt out at the beginning as well as a contractual obligation that, if any allegation of misconduct is made against any collaborator, they must agree to cooperate with any ensuing enquiries.

Having the correct procedures in place with the relevant documentation as outlined in the previous paragraph is all very well but, unless there is a robust system of monitoring in place, then we may be whistling in the wind. Clearly within universities, medical schools, and hospitals this should be done within divisional structures with the research supervisor reporting to the head of department and then to the divisional head. Such reportings need to be supported by regular unannounced visits or vivas, where the research student and supervisor are subject to "external" scrutiny. It must also be clear to all what the institution's policy is for investigating and managing any allegations of misconduct.

Research ethics committees

Just as research supervisors need training in research methodology and supervision, so research ethics committees need appropriate training so that they can detect loopholes in project submissions that might lead to perpetration of dishonesty. Furthermore local research ethics committees (LRECs) have a responsibility under the International Conference in Harmonisation (ICH) Agreement on Good Code of Practice to approve researchers as well as research protocols.[11] Whilst many LRECs do interview the research worker on a regular basis, problems obviously arise with the globalisation of research, multicentred trials, and collaborative projects. Multicentred research ethics committees (MRECs) cannot really know whether each investigator is properly schooled in research ethics or indeed is the appropriate person to undertake the submitted protocol.[12,13] Indeed, in the previous edition of this book and in the Edinburgh Consensus Statement Publication, Wells[12] described how two general practitioners fabricated LREC approval and how this could have been prevented. As Povl Riis wrote in his 1994 article on "Prevention and management of fraud in Theory": "Ethics and honesty/dishonesty are concepts of societies as a whole and not confined to the health sciences."[2] He also suggested that the presence of a majority (by one) of lay members on seven regional research ethics committees and on the central committee (by two) had proved indispensable. He further stated:

In the Danish control system for scientific dishonesty within the health services the chairman is a high court judge, and the secretary also is a lawyer, but the members are scientists representing medicine, pharmacy and dentistry. When the system was established it was foreseen that lay membership would be a part of the ultimate system, following a planned revision after 2–3 years. When the necessary definitions and analytic procedures have been laid down, it should be no more difficult for lay people to participate in the control process than in the research ethics committees.

The practicalities of introducing such a system in the UK are profound as are the resource implications.

The fact that in the UK the proposals for the new-style General Medical Council (GMC)[14] will comprise many more lay members than in the past attests to the pressures from society, an increasingly sophisticated and better educated public, and a radical change in attitudes to the medical and scientific communities with the acknowledgement that traditional "paternalism" is dead and gone.

Role of editors and peer review

The ability of editors and the peer review process to uncover research misconduct is controversial. Riis (1994) states that, "Editors have few opportunities both in theory and practice to detect and to prevent fraud." However, Farthing[15] writing six years later in the year 2000, has a more optimistic view, which may reflect the much higher profile of the problem and therefore the will to find solutions.

Whilst the peer review process is deemed hightly desirable and is meant to detect weaknesses in design and execution, most research misconduct has only come to light through the offices of "whistleblowers". However, the infamous Pearce paper on embryo implantation was not peer reviewed and the editor of the journal was himself a gift author;[9] the second paper deemed fraudulent was peer reviewed, and also reviewed by a statistician and a statistical report received, and it had also been through the LREC. With the gift of hindsight it was obvious that the number of patients reported to have been studied with this particular condition was highly unlikely given the catchment area of the investigator.[9] However, although stringent peer review may detect plagiarism and redundancy of publications, the downside of the peer review process is that the reviewers may themselves be guilty of misconduct by plagiarism of ideas or data or failing to declare conflicts of interest, including competitive grant funding in the area of research in question, as well as financial interests such as external consultancy remuneration.

Indeed, editors themselves are not immune from research misconduct with records of fabricated papers, introducing review bias, and a range of inbuilt prejudices.[15] However, the relatively recent establishment of the Committee on Publication Ethics (COPE) has been a force for good, where discussion of the issues of prevention are regularly debated.[16,17]

In the 1995 report from the independent committee of inquiry into the circumstances surrounding the publication of two articles in the *British Journal of Obstetrics and Gynaecology*, a series of "editorial" recommendations were made to aid in the of prevention of future fraudulent research papers.[9] Amongst many recommendations were the following.

Firstly no article should be accepted without a letter of submission signed by all authors, including confirmation that they understood the requirements for authorship and that journals must make these criteria absolutely transparent, in line with the International Committee of Medical Journal Editors (ICMJE) guidelines. Furthermore, they felt that consideration should be given to requesting that each author's role and area of responsibility is clearly specified in the letter of submission. This did not occur with the submission of the embryo implant case report. As discussed earlier, editors should feel free to request sight of raw data, and submission of a paper would include agreement that, if required such raw data would be provided. Indeed, it might be desirable to undertake random requests for raw data so that authors were aware that such verification was taking place. Thus, the ability to request raw data might detect fraud, whilst random requests might act as a deterrent.

The issue of "hawks" and "doves" as referees could partly be dealt with by the authors themselves suggesting appropriate referees, to be used at the discretion of editors, as well as authors indicating referees that they would not wish their paper to be sent to. It is also paramount that the referee be allocated by an editor who has no connection with the submitted article, either as an author or through the institution in which he or she works. If this had happened the fraudulent Pearce articles might never have seen the light of day. All papers being considered for publication with any statistical content should be reviewed by a statistician, and journals must allocate adequate resources for this to happen; if statistical queries are raised, the statistician must review the revisions prior to acceptance. Statisticians must also have a place at the editorial board table.

The embryo transplant paper was never refereed and two of the authors worked in an editorial capacity for the *British Journal of Obstetrics and Gynaecology*. The enquiry concluded that case reports should be dealt with using the standard operating system in a similar way to full papers and short reports, and must be refereed.

The enquiry then considered the system that should be in place when an editor is an author, or has an interest, or is associated with the authors, and concluded that a clear system must be in place with written documentation indicating the processes whereby such papers are dealt with. Clearly the process has to be entirely independent of the editor concerned. Therefore an independent editor must select the appropriate referees and deal with the manuscript, and the interested editor should never be present during any discussion at editorial meetings.

Many of these good practices are of course in place with many journals (but by no means all), and some of the enquiry's recommendations were peculiar to the *British Journal of Obstetrics and Gynaecology*. Of course there is no "evidence" that good editorial practices and good peer review processes will indeed be effective. This evidence needs to be acquired. The lessons to be learnt from the Pearce affair were also discussed in an editorial in the *BMJ* by Lock.[18]

Whistleblowers

A whistleblower is a person who is aware that misconduct is occurring and responds accordingly. Data concerning the prevalence of whistleblowers around the globe are difficult to obtain. Wilmshurst[19] in 1977 listed a series of instances when the UK employers (usually academics within universities) either failed to take seriously, or to make public, actions regarding allegations of or the uncovering of research misconduct. It makes depressing reading.

Frank Wells[12] discusses the role of whistleblowers citing the Pearce case as well as that of Fairhurst (Chapter 5), but in that article does not discuss his/her protection. Usually whistleblowers in any arena have a bad time, often being either disregarded, dismissed, suspended, pilloried, shamed, or threatened by peers or managers.[20] The most recent example (although not in the research arena) was the anaesthetist who blew the whistle on the results of paediatric heart surgery at the Bristol Royal Infirmary; he subsequently resigned and went to Australia to get another job. It is to be hoped that this will not happen in the future in the UK since, as of July 1999, the new 1998 Public Interest Disclosure Act provides some protection for whistleblowers. However, more importantly, as Frank Wells points out,[12] the hostile environment that whistleblowers find themselves in will only be improved when a stronger attitude of intolerance is shown towards research misconduct. This has also recently been enforced by the GMC in various publications[21] including "Good Medical Practice" outlining the professional duties of doctors to uphold the integrity of the medical profession. Of course the GMC has no jurisdiction over non-medically qualified scientists. Both the GMC and the Royal Colleges have a duty of care towards patients and, in the interest of patient safety and to maintain confidence in scientific research, whistleblowers must be given support and protection where appropriate. Donald Irvine, President of the GMC has stated, "Where doctors are implicated in research misconduct, decisive GMC action will follow. Doctors found guilty of serious professional misconduct in relation to research can expect to be erased from the medical register unless there are compelling mitigating circumstances."[22]

Allocation of resources for research

There are several question marks over the legal validity of the screening and investigation procedures designed to investigate research misconduct as discussed elsewhere in this volume. Thus many questions remain unresolved. Does a researcher suspected of misconduct have a contractual obligation to participate in the investigating procedures? If not they should. Whilst employees of the pharmaceutical industry, device manufacturers, and the UK's MRC do, in the main this is not usually in place within the university system or the NHS.

However, all grant-giving organisations will in future expect transparent procedures to be in place in the UK. The Association of Medical Research Charities (AMRC) has stated that their member charities should include as part of their guidance to research applicants the following:[23]

In the rare event of scientific fraud occurring (the Charity) wishes to make it clear that it is the responsibility of the employing authority to investigate this. (The Charity) agrees to funding providing the employing authority can produce evidence that they have in place a procedure for dealing with scientific fraud. If a case of scientific fraud is suspected in the course of the research then (the Charity) should be notified and kept informed of further developments. At the initial stages of the inquiry (the Charity) would not normally suspend the grant. However, if adequate steps are not taken to proceed with the investigation (the Charity) will suspend the grant. If fraud is proven, (the Charity) will terminate the grant immediately. Indeed, the AMRC outlines a viable mechanism for dealing with accusation of scientific fraud and states that it would probably contain the following elements;

1   A guidance document or code of practice on standards of professional behaviour.
2   Provisions for induction and training of staff.
3   Agreed arrangements for monitoring the process.
4   Regulation and procedures for handling allegations.
5   Fair procedures and appropriate protection for both the accused (respondent) and the "whistle-blower" (complainant).

The AMRC's statements are helpful but are not as robust as those within the pharmaceutical industry, where a monitoring and auditing system has long been in place (see below), despite the questions relating to the legality of such procedures.[24] Whilst grant-giving bodies such as the MRC have moved forward, a recent survey by the Council of Heads of Medical Schools in the UK revealed that universities have only belatedly begun tackling these issues.

Last year, the NHS has finally responded with the publication of a consultation document: the draft document *Research governance framework for health and social care*.[25] This sets out standards, delivery mechanisms, and monitoring arrangements for all research within the NHS in England and Wales. It also includes collaborative projects with other parties such as universities, charities, research councils, and the pharmaceutical industry. Dr Elizabeth Clough, Deputy Director of Research and Development for the Trent region in the UK and a member of the steering group who developed the framework, said; "There were two main imperatives for developing the framework. First it sets out standards and mechanisms to protect the needs, rights, well-being and safety of research participants. Second, the recommendations are designed to promote excellent quality research and on the flipside to prevent less good practice."

The framework makes the contents of study participants key to how research should be conducted stating, "The rights, safety and well-being of participants must be the primary consideration of any research study" (Box 17.1).

Monitoring and audit

In 1995 in response to an editorial[18] written in the *BMJ* by Stephen Lock concerning the fraudulent publications in the *British Journal of Obstetrics and Gynaecology*, Iain Chalmers and Muir Gray, both members of the NHS Research and Development Directorate, and Trevor Sheldon of the NHS Centre for Reviews and Development[26] agreed that national mechanisms must be in place to reassure the public that activities of the research community can, when necessary, be audited.

Box 17.1 Research governance framework for health and social care: the governance framework's recommendations

- Ethics
  - The rights, safety, and well-being of participants must be the primary consideration in any research study.
  - All research involving patients, users, and carers, or volunteers, or their data or material, must be reviewed independently to ensure it meets ethical standards.
  - Patient's data must be protected.
  - Research should reflect the diversity of the population.

- Science
  - Research that duplicates other work unnecessarily or that is not of sufficient quality to contribute something useful to existing knowledge is unethical.
  - All health and social care research should be subjected to rigorous review by recognised experts.

- Information
  - There should be free access to information on research and on its findings, once these have been subjected to appropriate scientific review.
  - Researchers should aim to publish their work and open it to critical review in the scientific press.
  - Studies involving direct contact with patients, users, and carers, or the public, should provide accessible accounts of the research.

- Health and safety
  - The safety of research participants and staff must be given priority at all times.
- Finance
  - Financial probity and compliance with the law and with the rules laid down by the Treasury for the use of public funds are as important in research as in any other area.

Dews and Vandenburg,[27] as long ago as 1991, in a letter to the *BMJ* entitled "Preventing fraud", drew attention to the part that good practice has played within the pharmaceutical industry.[28] The main thrust of good clinical practice is to protect the research subject and confirm the veracity of the research data. The elements of good clinical and research practice (GCP) have been enshrined within the many documents and legalities of the Food and Drug Administration (FDA), in the USA,[29] which were brought to Europe by the guidelines issued by the Committee for Proprietary Medical Products.[30]

Within the pharmaceutical and medical devices industries the responsibility for the veracity of the research data lies with the investigator(s) and the monitors. Monitors must validate by comparing the research data written in case report form with the clinical patient records and raw laboratory data. In time pharmaceutical companies operating within the GCP framework must have at least one tier of auditors to audit the performance of investigators and monitors. In the USA the FDA has a team of compliance officers who check data validity.[31] As Dews and Vandenberg wrote, "It is this typically American attitude of checks and balances that maximises the chance of detecting fraud in American pharmaceutical research." Furthermore, the FDA publishes a "blacklist" of researchers who have not met audit standards but, unlike the situation in Europe, it also has the power to institute change. We must also believe that the more recent advent of GCP in the UK and the rest of Europe will increase both detection and prevention of misconduct in research.

In the UK at present the only recourse is to the GMC, which of course has no jurisdiction over non-medically qualified scientific research workers. Europe still does not have any specific laws and, as Dews and Vandenburg wrote in 1991,[27] "no government undertook audit, with the exception of Greece, which has two auditors, and the only other country intending to audit was France, although no definitive audit had occurred". Today in the new millennium, ten years later, despite all the publicity, the situation is not much different. At this time in many countries in Europe, excluding the Nordic countries, there is no external audit body to monitor, and local efforts within individual research institutions is patchy.

Along with others,[31] it is difficult not to conclude that the pharmaceutical industry was doing much more to prevent misconduct and fraud in medical research than the many academic institutions and the NHS. Many researchers within the latter organisations can be scathing at worst or suspicious at best about the veracity of research sponsored by the industry compared with research sponsored by the traditional grant-giving bodies within academic institutions and the NHS. Maybe we should all be much more humble and learn their lessons, a view also expressed by others.[32]

Since then, things have indeed moved on and, in October 1996, the UK Medicines Control Agency formed a division to ensure GCP and to monitor compliance inspections and enforcement.

Parafraud

In an interesting letter to the *BMJ*[33] Hillman lists practices some of which currently do not lie under the umbrella of fraud and misconduct in research, which he defines as "parafraud". He lists the following:

- authors not publishing results that do not support hypotheses;
- authors not doing crucial control experiments;
- authors claiming authorship of papers towards which they have not made any contribution;

- authors leaving out some results of experiments arbitrarily;
- referees recommending rejection of papers for publication without specifying reasons and relevant refrences, or rejecting work that may yield results throwing into doubt the value of their own work;
- referees recommending that grants not be given to fund research by competitors;
- authors misquoting other authors deliberately;
- referees not reading manuscripts or submissions for grants with sufficient attention to assess them seriously;
- authors not answering questions at meetings or in correspondence;
- authors ignoring findings inimical to, or preceding, their own;
- authors being unwilling to discuss their own published research.

He also concludes that the extent and impact of these practices in the body of research are unknown but may be extensive.

Motivation and pressures that may have a role in research misconduct

Pressure to publish

In the UK the relatively recent introduction of the peer reviewed rating of research, the Research Assessment Exercise (RAE) within academic institutions and the consequent effect on the allocation of resources brings its own new scrutinies and pressures on research performance. Furthermore, the number of publications rather than any inherent assessment of quality is often used in NHS and academic appointment committees, so that financial pressure becomes inherent in these processes. Until the quantity issue is replaced by quality, this will remain undesirable, and possibly a pressure towards research misconduct.[34]

Whilst pressure to publish may well be the commonest cause, most investigations into research misconduct have rarely examined the motivation in depth. Scientific success is often achieved by the prolific output of research papers and this can have general knock-on effects including the following: academic promotion, discretionary points and merit awards leading to higher salaries, lucrative "consultancies", tenure of appointment, and increased research grant income. Of course in order to respond to these pressures, the "salami" approach to publication may be employed, resulting in multiple publications on virtually the same subject.

In the UK many medical researchers also undertake onerous clinical duties for the NHS and thus their time itself is very pressurised, which in itself may lead to research misconduct. As Forbes wrote,[35] "The overt signs of a researcher on the fast track are the number of publications in a very short space of time." He cites the Darsee affair, when 18 research manuscripts and about 100 other reports appeared in four years. Forbes also concludes that other high profile examples may have resulted from pressure to publish:

1974: William Summerlin, Sloan Kettering Institute – faking skin transplants.

1977: Robert Gullis, Birmingham University – faked research results for PhD and 11 papers.

1981: Michael Briggs, Deakin University, Australia – forged data on oral contraceptives.

1985: Robert Slutsky, University of California – 137 papers in seven years (48 questionable and 12 fraudulent).

1993: Roger Pauson, St Luc's Hospital, Montreal – falsified data on breast cancer trials.

Despite all this, however, Rennie, writing in the *BMJ* in 1998,[36] believes that we should all stop whingeing about the awful pressures of "publish or perish", as he thinks that we should stop being led astray by pretending that we know the motives when we can only speculate! He says that we have little credible evidence on what motivates misconduct or indeed, on the other hand, what motivates the conduct of honest equally stressed colleagues. A good point! He cites, "laziness, desire for fame, greed or an inability to distinguish right from wrong", and says there is an urgent need to encourage investigation in this area, including confidential experimental audits.[37]

Financial pressures

These are easier to identify and have clearly been a major pressure in several notable instances. This may often be a problem when the pharmaceutical industry is involved, when investigators receive payment in relationship to the number of patients recruited to the protocols, the number who are followed up, and who undergo continuing evaluation. However, as described earlier, the industry has better control over this with its systems of checks and balances. Of course, the industry is hugely motivated to prevent research misconduct. A company loses on average £650 000 (US $1m) a day in delay on registering a new drug. As Lars Breimer pointed out:[38]

Conducting a trial to good clinical practice standards costs about £20 000 (US $32 000) a patient. Thus if a 25-patient study has to be repeated and 100 days are lost a company can lose over £1m (US $1.6m); in the case of a 400-patient study requiring two years from start to finish it can lose about £500m (US $800 m). In addition, the reputation of the company is at stake. In the UK companies hand over the evidence to the institution where the person works and lets it act in the investigation, detection and outcome. If officers of medical schools or district general hospitals were to find themselves facing a bill of £500m plus legal costs, they would soon devise a fair and efficient system of investigating alleged misconduct.

Forbes[35] quotes other examples where money was the main motivation. Other cases with a financial motive include:

- JP Sedgwick, High Wycombe, UK – a family doctor in an antihypertensive trial; 121 records forged.

- 1988: VA Siddiqui, Durham, UK – faked data from an antidepressant trial.
- 1990: K Francis, Coventry – faked records in an antibiotic trial.
- 1991: S Kumar, Hornchurch – faked records in a hypertension trial.
- 1991: L Pandit, Wimbledon – faked records in trial of CAOD.
- 1991: D Latta, Glasgow – faked records in a hypertension trial.

Duff[39] also drew attention to other not so commonly cited potential causes as quoted below:

- New factors necessitate a change in research management.
- Globalisation of research activity makes it impossible to assess reliability through personal knowledge of others in the same field.
- Developments, such as bibliometrics, the research assessment exercise, and the link between research success and promotion, demand a stream of research publications.
- The expectation of institutions to generate income from their intellectual property (IP) has increased.
- Computer-based data acquisition, record-keeping, and display technologies increase the scope for falsification.

A strong case exists for all institutions to adopt the highest standards of record-keeping. The 1996 *International agreement on trade-related aspects of intellectual property* (TRIPs) recommends bound, consecutively-numbered notebooks, with numbered pages that are read and signed regularly by an independent scientist. In practice, there are many benefits beyond the securing of IP: diligent record-keeping, better project planning; a permanent and defensible record; a strong deterrent to falsification; early detection of irregularities; easier confirmation of veracity. Adopting TRIPs-compatible standards is a practical move, available to all research institutions, towards reducing fraudulence in science.

Illness

Documentation in this area is not good but in the absence of any other motivation it seems reasonable to conclude, given the prevalence of psychological morbidity and psychiatric illness within the general population, that this must be a relevant factor.

The way forward for the UK: lessons from elsewhere

As stated earlier, the Darsee affair was 30 years ago, and it is now over 12 years since Stephen Lock, the then editor of the *BMJ*, published the results of a personal survey "Misconduct in medical research: does it exist in Britain?"[40] Lock indeed concluded that it did and that urgent action should be taken to prevent the problem by establishing an organisation similar to the then Office of Scientific Integrity (OSI) in the USA, in order to alleviate professional and public alarm. In 1998, again writing in the *BMJ*, and later in 2000, Drummond Rennie of the Institute for Health Policy Studies in the USA and then a deputy editor of *JAMA* felt not much had happened in the UK.[36,37] He is right. Although he said he attended a meeting in 1995 hosted by the *BMJ* to discuss the issue and a later meeting of COPE, he felt that the UK was far too parochial in its approach and was failing to learn from the lessons of the last 30 years in the USA. He said he first became aware of the problem when deputy editor of the *New England Journal of Medicine* (*NEJM*) in 1979, when he was involved in a serious case of research fabrication and plagiarism.[41] Interestingly the publicity surrounding several other cases, including Darsee, resulted in a reaction by US Congress with more than 12 congressional hearings, the first in 1983 under the then Congressman Al Gore. Joining forces with the American Bar Association, the American Association for the Advancement of Science set about trying to frame a response to the growing public perception that a huge problem existed and that science was riddled with research misconduct. In 1989 the federal regulations were issued governing research that was sponsored by the US Public Health Service, which charged institutions to put in place procedures to oversee the integrity of their research.

Rennie describes how over the years the OSI moved from a "scientific dialogue model" to a more "legal model", and was replaced by the Office of Research Integrity (ORI) following procedures of administrative law, so that investigations could be handled more quickly and would be less open to challenge. The Commission on Research Integrity reported in 1995,[42] extending its earlier definition, basing it on the principle of telling the truth and suggesting a "whistleblowers' bill of rights and responsibilities". At the time of writing (1998) many of the issues surrounding whistleblowers were unresolved, and Rennie said that the Commission's findings were "widely resisted by a scientific community that still has difficulty coming to terms with the basic fact that, together with the privileges of a profession, come responsibilities." He concludes that the sooner the UK establishes a central body to oversee the issue the better.

Whilst COPE has done much to raise the profile of the issues, its members are understandably frustrated by the perceived inertia exhibited by the GMC, Royal Colleges, etc. The Edinburgh Consensus panel concluded that:

A national panel should be established – with public representation – to provide advice and assistance on request.

The panel might:

- develop and promote models of good practice for local implementation;
- provide assistance with the investigation of alleged research misconduct;
- collect, collate and publish information on incidents of research misconduct.

238

They continue: "We expect that this paper will be given the fullest possible dissemination by the sponsoring bodies and that the three Royal Colleges of Physicians and the Faculty of Pharmaceutical Medicine will convene at the earliest opportunity a meeting with the General Medical Council and appropriate partners to establish and consider the remit of the national panel."

In an angry polemic last year, three members of COPE berated the medical and scientific community for doing so little since Lock's first enquiry.[40]

As stated earlier the UK lags behind many other countries and most institutions have scant experience of dealing with allegations of research misconduct. The knowledge that robust systems are in place for detection and investigation should act as a powerful deterrent. Earlier in the USA the OSI developed an unfortunate relationship with the research communities mainly because it adopted a confrontational approach. The new ORI has developed a better partnership approach and subsequently there is more confidence in its procedures.

Evans[43] commenting on data from the ORI says:

There continue to be a number of investigators who are disciplined by the US Health Authorities and the (ORI). The most recent report by ORI presented an analysis of 150 scientific misconduct investigations which were completed between 1993 and 1997. The 150 investigations resulted in 76 findings of scientific misconduct and in 74 findings of no misconduct. Falsification was the most frequent type of misconduct that resulted in investigation, fabrication was second and plagiarism was third. There were about 1,000 allegations but no action was possible on two thirds of them. This was because the allegation did not contain sufficient specific information to proceed, or the whistle-blower was unknown, or unable or unwilling to provide additional data. Falsification and fabrication accounted for 86% of the investigations and 91% of the misconduct findings. Audits of studies in cancer and leukaemia suggested a very low incidence of misconduct in clinical trials (two instances over 11 years). It is not clear whether the audits were effective, since one institute passed the audit but was subsequently found to have problems.

The Nordic countries have also adopted a less confrontational approach and eschewed rigid definitions of research misconduct in favour of sound judgment. Their experience of seven years indicated that, of 68 allegations received, 47 were investigated and nine cases of research misconduct were identified. Whilst that may seem a small number, it only takes one case to undermine public and patient confidence in medical research.

As discussed earlier, in the UK the responsibilities must be with the employing authorities. Whilst such arrangements are in place in some organisations such as the MRC, many of the largest employers, for example the NHS and the universities, are light years behind. As George Radda, Chief Executive and Secretary, MRC has written:

Good research practice (GRP) is a key preventive strategy that underpins scientific integrity. GRP is concerned with the organisation of research; it governs the processes and conditions whereby studies are planned, carried out, monitored, recorded and reported. It permits the quality and integrity of data to be verified

239

and ensures that the fruits of research are applied and/or exploited appropriately. In essence, GRP is an attitude to work. The MRC has recently prepared detailed guidance on GRP for its staff. As with the MRC's procedure for dealing with allegations of scientific misconduct and guidelines on good clinical practice in clinical trials, we hope that this information will interest the broader research community and welcome feedback on our approach.[44]

As discussed earlier the NHS may find it easier to incorporate GRP into NHS research under the umbrella of Clinical Governance, than the universities.

The MRC has a stepwise approach (Box 17.2).[44,45]

Box 17.2 MRC's stepwise approach to scientific misconduct

- *Preliminary action* To determine whether the allegation falls within our definition of scientific misconduct.
- *Assessment* To determine whether there is *prima facie* evidence of scientific misconduct.
- *Formal investigation* To examine and evaluate all relevant facts to determine whether scientific misconduct has been committed and, if so, the responsible person(s) and seriousness of the misconduct.
- *Appeal*

Universities are more problematic since the medical schools within them are not autonomous and are answerable to their parent organisations. Any codes of practice in the arena of research misconduct would have to be agreed with the Committee of Vice Chancellors and Principals (now Universities UK) and adapted to the needs of individual universities. There is also the old argument about the disposition of responsibility when academic university employees undertake clinical research on honorary NHS contracts. Other medical organisations can and must play an important role. Thus, the medical royal colleges have published guidance in the area, particularly the Royal Colleges of Physicians (London) and Edinburgh.[45] They of course can exert a disciplinary role and can withdraw fellowships etc. from any found guilty of research misconduct. The Royal Societies (UK) and the recently founded Academy of Medical Sciences can also promote high standards and COPE, and the GMC likewise.

The GMC did indeed initiate a meeting of the representatives of the medical royal colleges and heads of medical schools to discuss the way forward, and out of this a committee was established. It has set in train a review of the 1991 Royal College of Physicians guidance[45,46] and with advice from others has a goal aimed at supplying transparent advice to universities and to the GMC itself. As part of this effort all UK medical schools were asked to submit their guidance and procedures within the framework of the GMC 1998 publication on *Good medical practice*.[21] As a result the GMC plans to produce a document on *Good practice in research* in the near future (GMC, 2001 personal communication).

Finally, the need for a separate overarching body to oversee good practice in medical research really requires an urgent airing at the highest level, with involvement of all interested parties. This can only be done by collaboration and dialogue together with representatives of patients and the laity, research institutions, royal medical colleges, hospitals, commercial laboratories, pharmaceutical companies, the law, politicians, and the GMC.

As a glance at any UK newspaper will reveal, public confidence in medicine, science, and scientific research is arguably at an all time low, and a concentrated effort to show that their concerns are taken seriously must be the best way forward and is of paramount importance for the good-standing of the scientific community.

The public and our patients

Last, but by no means least, we must involve our patients and the public in the debate. In an issue of the *BMJ* (12 April 1997), devoted to informed consent, comments were invited on the acceptable limits of informed consent in medical research. This resulted in a huge volume of correspondence and debate. Lisa Power, a health advocacy manager for the Terence Higgins Trust wrote, "There needs to be an understanding that giving patients or potential patients some say in the design and approval of trials is a positive process and not just a hoop to jump through. This involvement can stretch from trial design to writing information sheets and sitting on ethics committee." Often patients are only involved in research as altruistic volunteering subjects. At our peril do we ignore them or abuse them. Mostly they are never given feedback on the outcome of the research, or indeed are mostly not informed of the conclusions of research or even if it was ever completed. When research misconduct has occurred patients are most likely to learn this from the media. Thus, if in the UK we finally get to grips with the issue, involvement of lay people is absolutely essential.

We cannot expect patients to volunteer in a trusting relationship, that between researcher and subject, unless they have confidence in the processes and in the communication that must be at its heart. The more involvement of patients in all research arenas, be it grant-giving bodies, ethics committees, monitoring and auditing, and with a spirit of openness and trust the better. Whilst fraud and misconduct in medical research continues we are all losers. Within a healthy framework that discourages, prevents, detects, and metes out justice where appropriate, every one is a winner, there can be no losers.

Declarations of interest

The author was a member of the 1995 independent inquiry into the fraudulent articles published in the *British Journal of Obstetrics and Gynaecology*. She was also a member of the Edinburgh Consensus Panel on Fraud and Misconduct in Medical Research, 2000.

References

1 Riis P. Creating a national control system on scientific dishonesty within health sciences. In: Lock S, Wells F, eds. *Fraud and misconduct in medical research*. London: BMJ, 1996, pp.114–17.
2 Riis P. Prevention and management of fraud-in theory. *J Int Med* 1994;**235**:107–13.
3 Proceedings of the Royal College of Physicians of Edinburgh. *Consensus Statement. Fraud and misconduct in medical research* Suppl. No. 7, Jan 2000.
4 Institute of Medicine. *The responsible conduct of research in the health sciences*. Washington, DC: National Academy Press, 1989.
5 Evans I. Conduct unbecoming – the MRC's approach. *BMJ* 1998;**316**:1728–9.
6 Radda G. How should we prevent it. *Proc R Coll Physicians Edinb* 2000;**30**:25.
7 Kalichman MW, Friedman PJ. A pilot study of biomedical trainees' perceptions concerning research ethics. *Acad Med* 1992;**67**:769–75.
8 Sachs GA, Siegler M. Teaching scientific integrity and the responsible conduct of research. *Acad Med* 1993;**68**:871–5.
9 Royal College of Obstetricians and Gynaecologists. *Report of the independent inquiry into circumstances surrounding the publication of two articles in the British Journal of Obstetrics and Gynaecology*. London: RCOG, 1995.
10 Allen G. Raw data. *Nature* 1998;**339**:500.
11 Proceedings of the Fourth International Conference on Harmonisation. Appendix 7. *Guideline for good clinical practice*. Brussels, 1997.
12 Wells FO. Clinical research fraud and misconduct: how is it diagnosed? *Proc R Coll Physicians Edinb* 2000;**30**:13–17.
13 Carnell D. Doctor struck off for scientific fraud. *BMJ* 1996;**312**:400.
14 Beecham L. GMC urged to be more radical. *BMJ* 2000;**321**:725.
15 Farthing MJG. What is the role of peer review? *Proc R Coll Physicians Edinb* 2000;**30**:23.
16 Williams N. Editors seek ways to cope with fraud. *Science* 1997;**278**:1221.
17 Committee on Publication Ethics. *Annual Report 1999*. London: BMJ Publishing Group, 1999.
18 Lock S. Lessons from the Pearce affair: handling scientific fraud. *BMJ* 1995;**310**:547–8.
19 Wilmshurst P. The code of silence. *Lancet* 1977;**349**:567–9.
20 La Follette M. *Stealing into print*. Berkley: University of California Press, 1992, pp. 137–55.
21 General Medical Council. *Good medical practice*. London: GMC, 1998.
22 Irvine D. How should we respond? *Proc R Coll Physicians Edinb* 2000;**30**:24.
23 AMRC Position Statement.
24 Wells F. Fraud and misconduct in medical research. *Br J Clin Pharmacol* 1997;**43**:3–7.
25 Mayor S. New governance framework for NHS research aims to stop fraud. *BMJ* 2000; **321**:725.
26 Chalmers SI, Gray M, Sheldon T. Prospective registration of health care research would help. *BMJ* 1995;**311**:262.
27 Dews IM, Vandenburg MJ, Preventing fraud. *BMJ* 1991;**302**:907.
28 Department of Health. *Good laboratory practice. The United Kingdom compliance programme*. London: DoH, 1989.
29 United States Code of Federal Regulations. Title 21: Sections 50, 56 and 312.
30 Committee for Proprietary Medical Products. *Good clinical practice*. Brussels: CPMP, 1991.
31 Brown L. Pharmaceutical industry follows guidelines on conduct of research. *BMJ* 1998;**317**:1590.
32 Thomas G. Preventing fraud. *BMJ* 1991;**302**:660.
33 Hillman H. Some aspects do not fall within remit of bodies examining fraud. *BMJ* 1998; **317**:1591.
34 Skinner A. Quality not quantity in NHS research output should be used as a yardstick of ability. *BMJ* 1998;**317**:1590.
35 Forbes CD. Why does it happen? *Proc R Coll Physicians Edinb* 2000;**30**:22–3.
36 Rennie D. Dealing with research misconduct in the United Kingdom. *BMJ* 1998;**316**:1726–33.
37 Rennie D. Why is action needed? *Proc R Coll Physicans Edinb* 2000;**30**:22.
38 Breimer L. Fair and efficient systems of investigating alleged misconduct can be devised. *BMJ* 1998;**317**:1590.
39 Duff G. The researcher perspective. *Proc R Coll Physicians Edinb* 2000;**30**:26.

40 Lock S. Misconduct in medical research: does it exist in Britain? *BMJ* 1988;**297**:1531–5.
41 Broad W, Wade N. *Betrayal of the truth*. Simon and Schuster, 1982.
42 Commission on Research Integrity. *Integrity and misconduct in research*. Report of the Commission on Research Integrity to the Secretary of Health and Human Services, the House Committee on Commerce and the Senate Committee on Labor and Human Resources. Rockville, MD: US Department of Health and Human Services, Public Health Service. 1995.
43 Evans SJW. How common is it? *Proc R Coll Physicians Edinb* 2000;**30**:9–11.
44 Medical Research Council. *MRC policy for inquiry into allegations of scientific misconduct*. London, MRC, 1997 (Ethics Series).
45 Royal College of Physicians. *Fraud and misconduct in medical research*. London: RCP, 1991.
46 Chantler C, Chantler S. Deception: difficulties and initiatives. *BMJ* 1998;**316**:1731–2.

18: Research misconduct: an editor's view

MICHAEL FARTHING

In the world of biomedical publishing, many editors like myself are part-timers. Our experience of journal editing and publishing may be extremely limited before we take on the job, yet we have a major responsibility as custodians of the biomedical literature. We bring our academic expertise, our experiences as authors and peer-reviewers, and some may have edited books and other publications, but as a group we are vulnerable. We have to learn our trade from other editors, short courses and personal experience. I felt most vulnerable, however, when I had to deal with dishonesty, namely publication and research misconduct.

I became editor of *Gut*, a specialist journal for gastroenterology and hepatology in 1996.[1] In my first year we detected redundant publication, "salami slicing" (publishing a study piecemeal when a single, high quality paper would have been preferable), outright plagiarism, and papers being submitted without the knowledge or consent of co-authors. Compared with the major cases of fraud that have come to light in recent years, these were relatively minor offences and all were detected prior to publication. Retractions were therefore not required and no author faced public disgrace. However, they raised important questions for me as an editor and I hope for the individuals concerned when their actions were discovered. I found it difficult, for instance, to know how far to go in investigating the alleged misconduct. When a reviewer drew my attention to serious plagiarism in an article submitted to the journal, should I have carried out an extensive examination of the author's other publications to determine whether this was a habit or a one-off? Should I have reported this to anyone? Should I have discussed the problem with another editor or the appropriate regulatory agency for the country concerned (this was not a paper from the UK)? Should I punish the authors in some way such as by refusing to consider further papers for the journal say for a period of three years, or should I reject the paper, just forget about it, and do nothing more?

There is a feeling amongst editors and some investigators that research misconduct has become more frequent during the last two decades. It is difficult to be certain whether this perceived increase is a true increase in the number of misdemeanours *committed*, but there is no doubt that the number of serious cases of research misconduct that have been *detected* has increased during this period. Stephen Lock, a past editor of the *British Medical Journal*, has documented known or suspected cases of research misconduct in the UK, USA, Australia, Canada, and in other countries.[2] In the UK many of the cases involve fabrication of clinical trial data most commonly by general practitioners although hospital clinicians have been guilty of similar offences. Fraud in laboratory experimentation appears less common, although there have been a number of notorious cases in the USA and UK when the results of laboratory experiments have been fabricated, falsified, or misrepresented. Thus the climate has changed. The days are gone when an editor can ignore publication and research ethics. Merely rejecting a suspect paper is no longer acceptable. Editors must fully engage with the world of biomedical science by ensuring that they fulfil their duties at all levels of editorship.

It was these demands on editors and the lack of an advisory group or independent agency to deal with alleged cases of research misconduct that resulted in the establishment of the Committee on Publication Ethics (COPE) in 1997.[3] This informal group of editors has grown and now represents a substantial proportion of biomedical journals in the UK. Although its function is purely advisory, it has considered more than 100 possible cases of research and publication misconduct and has produced guidelines on *Good publication practice* (see Appendix). The working of the committee will be discussed in more detail later in this chaper.

Publication ethics and the editor

Investigators, research students, authors, peer-reviewers, and journal editors must operate within an ethical framework that is transparent and has principles that are understood and accepted by all players in the biomedical research community. Publication ethics is a broad term embracing the many processes involved in the conduct of research and its publication.[4] The spectrum ranges from the most serious types of research fraud to the criteria required for authorship and the failure to declare *conflicts of interest* in research publications. Editors in addition must be concerned with ethical issues associated with the reviewing process and the legitimacy of product advertising in their journals. For the author and editor, publication ethics can be considered under two major categories, research integrity and publication integrity.

Research integrity

This must be uppermost in the investigator's mind during the conception, design, and execution of a research study. It is a multistep process and ethical considerations occur throughout. At the initiation of the research process there should be a protocol that has been reviewed and approved by all

Box 18.1 Research misconduct

- Errors of judgment
  - Inadequate study design
  - Bias
  - Self-delusion
  - Inappropriate statistical analysis

- Misdemeanours ("trimming and cooking")
  - Data manipulation
  - Data exclusion
  - Suppression of inconvenient facts

- Fraud
  - Fabrication
  - Falsification
  - Plagiarism

contributors and collaborators. Research integrity therefore covers study design, collection and collation of results, data analysis and presentation. Failure to ensure integrity in any of these components can amount to research misconduct. However, this will form a continuum ranging from errors of judgment (that is, mistakes made in good faith) to what have been regarded as minor misdemeanours, so called "trimming and cooking", through to blatant fraud, usually categorised as fabrication, falsification, and plagiarism (Box 18.1).

Publication integrity

This begins with the writing of the paper. Common examples of failure to meet acceptable standards include inappropriate or "gift" authorship, redundant (or duplicate) publication when all or a substantial part of the work has been published previously, and plagiarism in which text is "lifted" directly from another publication. Full declaration of any conflicts of interest is vital to encourage authors to ensure balance in their discussion and conclusions, and to facilitate peer review. Conflicts include direct or indirect financial support from the study, consultancy agreement with a study sponsor, the holding of any patents relating to the study, and any other mechanisms by which financial benefit might accrue as a result of publication of the study. Authors should declare all such associations, and it is the responsibility of editors to ensure that these are clearly detailed in any publication. The tendency to attempt to identify "the minimal publishable unit" sometimes referred to as "salami-slicing" should be discouraged.

Editors have other ethical concerns particularly about the quality of peer review and conflicts of interest that might arise in the review process. It is essential that editors reinforce to peer-reviewers the need to observe the rules of confidentiality; in many respects the relationship between an editor (and the reviewer) and an author is similar to the doctor–patient relationship. Additional concerns relate to sponsored supplements to the journal and the influence that advertising by the biomedical industry and others might have on journal content.

What is research and publication misconduct?

Misconduct can be committed at any point along the research–publication continuum. Although investigators/authors are usually considered to be the main perpetrators of research and publication misconduct, any person involved in the process is a potential offender. Peer-reviewers may fail to declare conflicts of interest when reviewing a manuscript or research proposal.[5] COPE has considered a number of cases in which authors have complained about the quality of reviews and expressed concerns that the individual concerned may be using anonymity to hide behind an inappropriately destructive report because of an unhealthy wish to retard the progress of the manuscript and the author's research group. COPE has also seen examples where reviewers have abused the confidentiality entrusted to them and plagiarised the material or ideas contained within a paper or grant proposal.

Similarly editors may breach ethical standards particularly with respect to conflicts of interest. In the same way that authors are now required to declare competing interests, notably commercial affiliations, financial interests, and personal connections, so must editors. Editors can influence the chances of acceptance or rejection of a paper by selecting "hawks" or "doves" to review the paper. Editors have also abused their position and published their own fabricated papers, sometimes bypassing the usual peer-review process.

There are a multitude of misdemeanours that are commonly brought together under the headings of research and publication misconduct.[4] At the milder end of the spectrum there are sins of omission; an example would be when experimental design is inadequate to answer the questions raised in the study. Similarly the inappropriate use of statistical analyses may produce inaccuracies both in the final results and in the conclusions reached. This occurs through ignorance but also by intent. Selective presentation of results through data suppression or exclusion may similarly influence the research findings to produce apparently "clear cut" results but that are at the same time misleading. It is always easier to write a paper when everything fits neatly together! Finally the major offences of fabrication, falsification, and plagiarism constitute outright research fraud. It is these major crimes that have been picked up avidly by the daily press, and in the UK have resulted in doctors being struck off by the GMC.

Some scientists argue that even overtly fraudulent research is not as dangerous as many would like to have us believe, since others will repeat

247

the work and, if it is found to be false, will eventually put the record right and make this clear in the biomedical literature. I would argue that this "soft line" makes a complete nonsense of the fundamental premise on which scientific research is based, namely "honesty". In addition, it is a deplorable waste of time and resources to prove that fraudulent research is false. In addition, damage can be done before the truth about falsified research eventually comes to light as illustrated by a paper published in 1993 in the *British Medical Journal* that was subsequently retracted last year after five years' exposure in the public domain.[6] This paper was of sufficient public health importance to change the delivery of services in a region of the UK.

There are instances when there are no questions about a way in which a piece of research was conducted but, in the process of preparing the manuscript for publication and the manner in which the paper is presented to a journal, the authors commit publication misconduct. A common problem centres on authorship. It is now well recognised that individuals' names often appear on a paper whose contribution to the work is questionable, so-called "gift authorship". The Vancouver Group of Editors has published guidelines on what constitutes authorship, which, for example, would exclude a widely held custom to include the head of department as a "courtesy" (Box 18.2).[7] There is now a move away from *authorship* towards *contributorship*, in which each individual outlines at the end of the paper their individual contributions to the work. There would also be a *guarantor* who would take overall responsibility for the veracity of the paper.[8] Disputes between authors are also common, ranging from failure to get approval from all authors before the final manuscript is submitted to a journal, to changes in authorship or the order of authors during manuscript revisions.

Some authors still submit papers simultaneously to two journals (dual submission) while others attempt to identify "the minimal publishable

Box 18.2 Authorship*

- Authorship credit should be based only on substantial contributions to:
  - conception and design or analysis and interpretation of data;
  - drafting the article or revising it critically for important intellectual content;
  - final approval of the version to be published.
- These conditions must all be met.
- Participation solely in the acquisition of funding or the collection of data does not justify authorship.
- General supervision of the research group is also not sufficient for authorship.

* From reference 7.

unit" sometimes referred to as "salami-slicing". Most editors would prefer to see a substantial manuscript containing a cohesive story rather than a string of minor contributions in a variety of different journals.

Failure to declare conflicts of interest is another aspect of publication misconduct. Conflicts include direct or indirect financial support from the study, consultancy agreement with a study sponsor, a holding of any patents relating to the study, and any other mechanisms by which financial benefits might accrue as a result of publication of the study. It has been said, "disclosure is almost a panacea".

Diagnosis of fraud

Serious research fraud is usually discovered during the formal audit or monitoring process of randomised controlled trials when all patients apparently recruited into the study cannot be accounted for from a search of independent medical records.[9] Fraudulent clinical trials have also been detected after publication, often when there are some unusual features to the study. Surprising, unexpected results emerging from an apparently, large single-centre study written up by a single author might attract attention. Published work may come into question when an investigator is found to have committed research misconduct and previously published fraudulent work is then revealed following a systematic review of the contents of the author's *curriculum vitae*. The other important route by which research fraud is detected is through a whistleblower, commonly a colleague in the same or a closely related department. Although there are many examples when whistleblowers have subsequently suffered more than the accused, there is now a firm legal framework to protect people in the workplace who become concerned about the behaviour of colleagues.

One of the most active, contemporary whistleblowers in the UK is Peter Wilmshurst, a consultant cardiologist in Shrewsbury. Wilmshurst wrote an article in the *Lancet* in 1997 entitled "The code of silence" in which he suggested that there were a number of cases of research misconduct in the UK that had not been adequately investigated or suppressed, perhaps by senior members of the profession.[10] One of the cases referred to anonymously in this report was finally brought before the Professional Conduct Committee of the GMC in November 2000; this resulted in the suspension of a Dr Anjan Banerjee, a surgeon from Halifax.[11,12] It took almost a decade for this case to be resolved despite the fact that many colleagues knew of the allegations for much of this period, and certain individuals, who had been willing to speak out, were silenced with the threat that their future career would be at stake. Peter Wilmshurst assembled the evidence and eventually the case was heard. Without his tenacity it is unlikely that Banerjee would have been required to face his misdemeanours nor would the medical literature have been corrected.

This sounds like a satisfactory ending to an otherwise sad story. However, a number of issues remain unresolved. As editor of the journal in which Banerjee published his fraudulent work I am responsible for issuing a retraction notice in the journal, a request that came promptly from the author following the GMC judgment. However, it is extremely difficult to effectively erase an article from the published literature since the November 1991 issue of *Gut* will remain on library shelves for many decades to come without any indication that the Banerjee paper is fraudulent. In addition we know that retracted papers continue to be cited after retraction almost invariably without reference to the falsehoods that are contained therein.[13] If publication of scientific material becomes solely electronic, only then will it be possible to erase a paper completely and put the record straight. Another issue is the delay that has occurred in bringing this case to the GMC. Intuitively most of us would believe that it would be preferable to solve a crime promptly to minimise the risk that further misdemeanours might be committed. Banerjee had already been suspended by his NHS Trust earlier in 2000 for, I understand, a totally different reason and has recently resigned from this post. Whether earlier resolution of the research misconduct case would have influenced this issue remains a matter for speculation.

Unfortunately the case does not rest here. Banerjee's supervisor at the time he produced the fraudulent work, Professor Tim Peters, also appeared before the GMC in early 2001, when he was administred for his role in the affair. Finally, and perhaps most important of all, what happened following the internal enquiry of the Banerjee case at King's College Hospital Medical School in 1991 will be determined. If Banerjee's work, as it is alleged, was found to be questionable at that time,[10] why did the Dean of the day not refer the case to the GMC immediately? Why was the *Gut* paper not retracted in 1991 and why did Banerjee's supervisor remain associated with the work when other collaborators withdrew their names from the paper?

We all have a responsibility to be vigilant about the quality of research with which we are directly or indirectly associated. If you have suspicions that a colleague may be producing research findings dishonestly, the most important first step is to ensure that you obtain evidence of your suspicions before reporting this to a senior colleague. In some instances it may be entirely appropriate to discuss this with the person concerned, particularly if you feel that the main problem is "trimming and pruning", which the individual may be pursuing out of ignorance. Similarly, if there are potential misdemeanours regarding publication ethics, such as dual submission or redundant publication, then these should be dealt with by open discussion. However, if the misdemeanours are of a more serious nature, such as fabrication or falsification of research data, then you must try to provide evidence of the misdemeanours before reporting to a higher authority. I have been approached by potential whistleblowers who have waited weeks or even several months to ensure that their suspicions are well founded. At this point you should discuss this with your head of department, although, if that individual is directly involved with the research, it may be more appropriate to discuss your concerns immediately with the head of the institution. At this point a preliminary inquiry should be performed along the lines described in the Royal College of Physicians Working Party Report[14] or as described in the Medical Research Council's document, which describes a procedure for inquiring into allegations of scientific misconduct within MRC units.[15]

Journal editors and reviewers also detect research and publication misconduct. In my experience as an editor of a specialist journal, sharp-eyed reviewers have drawn my attention to the majority of cases of misconduct that I have come across in the past three years. However, in almost every case there has been an element of serendipity about the discovery. For example, in one case of plagiarism that we have seen, I just happened, by chance, to send the manuscript to a reviewer whose papers had been plagiarised. How many other manuscripts have passed through the system and escaped detection because the reviewer did not have such an intimate knowledge of the text of related papers? Redundant publication and "salami-slicing" are again usually detected by expert reviewers who know their subject well. On several occasions, we have by chance sent a manuscript to a reviewer who had been sent a closely related and in some cases an identical manuscript by the same authors from another journal, simultaneously. In this case publication can be stopped but if the manuscript had been sent to another reviewer, who had not seen the closely related manuscript, then both manuscripts could have entered the public domain with inevitable redundancy. Thus, the detection of publication and research misconduct seems to carry with it a large element of chance and many editors of biomedical journals suspect that only a small proportion of misdemeanours are detected. It would appear that crime does pay! Diagnostic approaches would thus seem to be inadequate and, given the obvious limitations that a whistleblower, editor, or reviewer might have, perhaps we should focus our attention more on treatment and prevention.

Treatment of fraud

When serious fraud, such as fabrication of controlled clinical trial data, is detected, the person or persons concerned would be reported to the GMC. If a preliminary review of the evidence suggests that there were sufficient grounds to proceed, then the GMC would hold a full enquiry and, if the defendant is found guilty, this might result in exclusion from the Medical Register. For lesser crimes and those involving non-clinical scientists, a whistleblower or journal editor might refer the case to the head of the investigator's department or institution. Reporting an individual to the head of institution, however, might not necessarily produce satisfactory outcome, as there may be conflict of interest. For example, the senior author might be a prominent clinical academic within the institution and possibly even a personal friend of the Dean or Vice-chancellor. There are a

251

number of instances of alleged, serious research misconduct that have been "silenced" within the investigator's institution.[10] It is difficult to feel confident that internal inquiries into alleged research misconduct held "in camera" will reliably get at the truth, when for the institution there is so much to lose and little to gain.

Editors face some difficult issues when they suspect or detect research fraud. Once a journal has published a paper that is subsequently shown to be fraudulent or redundant, then the paper would be retracted and a notice to that effect published in the journal. This places the case in the public domain and the authors are exposed. In serious cases the editor may, in the case of clinical investigators, refer the matter to the GMC. A recent study has shown, however, that this does not stop the paper being cited in the literature for many years, usually without making any reference to the fabrication or falsification contained therein.[13]

It is, however, more difficult to know precisely how to act when research misconduct is suspected during the peer-review process before publication. The most common editorial response is to simply reject the manuscript. This is clearly unsatisfactory and one might argue that the editor has not fulfilled his/her duty as a custodian of the biomedical literature, since it is likely that the paper would merely be submitted to another journal. Some editors have taken a "hard line" and have placed sanctions on all authors who engage in redundant publication, such as by refusing to accept further submissions to the journal for a set period, say three years.[16] Editors who are members of the Committee for Publication Ethics[17] (COPE) have produced some guidelines on *Good publication practice* (available in the 1999 COPE Report[18] or on the COPE website www.publicationethics.org.uk), which set down a hierarchy of sanctions that editors may publish in their journals and use judiciously such that "the punishment fits the crime". These might range from a firm letter to the author pointing out the breach of publication ethics when it is felt that an error occurred through ignorance and not malintent, through to tougher sanctions such as limited access to the journal for a given period as described above, or ultimately to referral of the matter to the author's head of institution or directly to the GMC. The Royal College of Physicians, London and the MRC have produced guidance on the investigation and prevention of research misconduct.[14,15]

Prevention of fraud

Although it might be hoped that investigators would be less inclined to commit research and publication misconduct if they knew the chances of getting caught and punished were increased, ultimately the route to prevention must be through education and reaffirmation of the still widely held belief in the principle of *research honesty*. All students entering a period of research should not only receive instruction on research design, methodology, and laboratory techniques but also guidance on the fundamentals of research and publication ethics (Box 18.3). Research should be protocol driven, and contributors and collaborators should define their roles before the work is commenced. Any protocol changes should be discussed and agreed by all of the participants. Statistical advice should be sought, where appropriate, during the planning process, and it goes without saying that all studies involving human subjects should be submitted to an appropriate research ethics committee. There is a sense that at least some of the instances of research misconduct could have been avoided by closer supervision of the project. Supervisors can find themselves increasingly distanced from the laboratory bench or the patients in the clinic, which can make it difficult to check the veracity of the primary data. Review of research results should involve examination of the primary research record, which may be the laboratory record book or patient's medical notes. Impeccable record keeping is an essential component of good research.

Box 18.3 Can research and publication misconduct be prevented?

- Education
  - Research training
  - Research ethics
  - Publication ethics
- The research
  - Protocol driven
  - Establish contributors and collaborators
    - define roles
    - agree protocol
    - agree presentation of results
  - Define methodology for data analysis
    - statistical advice
  - Ethical approval
  - Project and personal licence (Home Office)
  - Supervision
    - guarantor
    - communication
    - ensure good clinical practice
    - record keeping
- The publication
  - Disclose conflict of interest
  - Disclose previous publications
  - Approval by **all** contributors
  - Submit to one journal at a time
  - Assume research data audit

The ethics of publication are as important as research ethics. All authors should see the final manuscript before submission and each sign the declaration confirming the originality of the work. An article should only be submitted to one journal at a time. Authors should disclose any potential conflicts of interest, particularly if the opinions expressed in the manuscript could be influenced by financial incentives through sponsors. Authors should also disclose the nature of any related publications that have been published recently or that are under consideration by another journal. There are times when it is entirely reasonable to publish some previously published data, but this should be done with the full knowledge of the editor and reviewers, so that a full assessment can be made as to the extent of any potential overlap. In the future, original research may be submitted to random audit prior to publication and it is therefore wise that authors assume that they may be asked to produce their primary data to support the work described in a manuscript.

The foundation of COPE and its role in dealing with misconduct

The Committee on Publication Ethics (COPE) began unpretentiously in 1997 with an informal meeting of a group of medical editors, all of whom had expressed concern about the lack of clear guidelines as to how to deal with breaches of research and publication ethics.[3] At this first meeting it was soon evident that the group had collectively dealt with the full spectrum of research misconduct. As editors we felt an intense sense of frustration because of our extremely limited powers to deal with research dishonesty.

COPE was therefore established as an editors' self-help group, providing a forum in which we could advise each other about the management of difficult cases. All cases are considered anonymously and the final responsibility for action would always remain with the reporting editor. COPE has continued to have only an advisory role to editors. It has no authority to investigate cases of alleged misconduct and has no powers to make judgments or punish offenders. However, it has considered more than 100 cases of possible misconduct in the last three years and has reported its experience in annual reports. In the COPE Report 2000[19] we list the biomedical journals that are now part of COPE and have produced a draft constitution to ensure sound management and governance of COPE in the future. The experience with COPE has convinced many of us that the current procedures available in the UK to deal with research misconduct are inadequate.[12] The GMC considers only the more serious cases of alleged misconduct by medical practitioners and thus another independent body is required to consider the broad spectrum of misdemeanours that might be committed by clinical and non-clinical investigators.

The future

The recent Banerjee case at the GMC illustrates a number of important deficiencies in the way in which we handle possible cases of research misconduct in the UK. Firstly, it is evident that it is relatively simple to fabricate data and get it published in a reputable medical journal. In the majority of cases it will be virtually impossible for reviewers and editors to identify fraudulent material. Detection in this case, and in many others, will almost always depend on the willingness of a vigilant whistleblower to speak out. As stated previously, there is little in it for the whistleblower, particularly when their comments fall on "deaf ears" or they are threatened with professional extinction. Secondly, the case demonstrates the potential weakness of the *internal enquiry*. Although it is unclear as to the location of the final resting place of the King's Banerjee Report, it is alleged that its findings were not in Banerjee's favour.[10] It then took almost a decade and the persistent efforts of an external whistleblower who had no conflicting interests to bring the case to the GMC. This cannot be regarded as a satisfactory state of affairs and will do nothing to reassure the public that the medical profession is still fit to self-regulate. The case also shows the importance of the role of the research supervisor as a custodian of research quality. When it was clear in 1991 that Banerjee's work was suspect, did he not withdraw his support and insist on an external review by the GMC?

This case, and indeed many others considered by COPE and probably others still in the GMC pipeline, convinces me that the procedures currently in place in the UK are inadequate to deal with many of the possible instances of research misconduct. COPE has campaigned for more than three years for an independent body to consider such cases.[20] Although many universities and medical schools have written guidance as to how to pursue an internal review, I have concerns that a lack of independence may not be facilitatory for an otherwise reluctant whistleblower and provide appropriate protection when required. In October 1999 a consensus conference was held at the Royal College of Physicians in Edinburgh on Misconduct in Biomedical Research. The consensus panel recommended that a National Panel should be established that would develop and promote models of good practice for local implementation, provide assistance with the investigation of alleged research misconduct, and collect, collate, and publish information on the incidence of research misconduct. Although discussions have taken place and a report is said to be in preparation, no clear action has as yet become apparent to those of us on the outside.[21] Even if such an advisory panel is established, will it really have the teeth to ensure that we do not have a rerun of the Banerjee case? I have my doubts. What COPE is proposing is not new. The USA, Nordic countries, and others have had external agencies in place to deal with alleged cases of research misconduct for almost 10 years;[22] why is the UK lagging behind? One is reminded of the fact that it took 20 years longer to establish Research Ethics Committees in Britain than it did in the USA!

Acknowledgements

Some of the material in this paper has been published previously in reference 4 with kind permission of the BMJ Publishing Group. I am especially grateful to all of the members of COPE who have provided such a stimulating environment in which many of the ideas and concepts contained in this paper have evolved. I am particularly indebted to Richard Smith and Richard Horton who have taught me so much about the principles and practice of editorship. I should also like to pay a personal tribute to Peter Wilmshurst who continues to be a thorn in the flesh of the medical profession for the very best of reasons.

References

1 Farthing MJG. Research misconduct. *Gut* 1997;**41**:1–2.
2 Lock S. Research misconduct: a résumé of recent events. In: Lock S, Wells F, eds. *Fraud and misconduct in medical research*, 2nd edn. London: BMJ Publishing Group, 1996, pp. 14–39.
3 Smith R. Misconduct in research: editors respond. *BMJ* 1997;**315**:201–2.
4 Farthing MJG. Ethics of publication. In: Hall GM, ed. *How to write a paper*. 2nd edn. London: BMJ Books, 1998.
5 Smith R. Peer review: reform or revolution? Time to open up the black box of peer review. *BMJ* 1997;**315**:759–60.
6 Bowie C. Was the paper I wrote a fraud? *BMJ* 1998;**316**:1755.
7 International Committee of Medical Journal Editors. Uniform requirements for manuscripts submitted to biomedical journals. *Ann Intern Med* 1997;**126**:36–47.
8 Smith R. Authorship: time for a paradigm shift? *BMJ* 1997;**314**:992.
9 Dyer C. Consultant struck off over research fraud. *BMJ* 1997;**315**:205.
10 Wilmshurst P. The code of silence. *Lancet* 1997;**349**:567–9.
11 Ferriman A. Consultant suspended for research fraud. *BMJ* 2000;**321**:1429.
12 White C. Plans for tackling research fraud may not go far enough. *BMJ* 2000;**321**:1487.
13 Budd JM, Sievert ME, Schultz TR. Phenomena of retraction. *JAMA* 1998;**280**:296–7.
14 Working Party. *Fraud and misconduct in medical research. Causes, investigation and prevention.* London: Royal College of Physicians, 1991.
15 Medical Research Council. *Policy and procedure for inquiring into allegations of scientific misconduct.* MRC Ethics Series, Surrey: Aldridge Print Group, 1997.
16 Doherty M. The misconduct of redundant publication. *Ann Rheum Dis* 1996;**55**:783–5.
17 Williamson A, White C, eds. *The COPE Report 1998*. London: BMJ Publishing Group, 1998.
18 White C, ed. *The COPE Report 1999. Annual Report of the Committee on Publication Ethics.* London: BMJ Books, 1999.
19 White C, ed. *The COPE Report 2000. Annual Report of the Committee on Publication Ethics.* London: BMJ Books, 2000.
20 Farthing MJG. An editor's response to fraudsters. *BMJ* 1998;**316**:1729–31.
21 Farthing M, Horton R, Smith R. UK's failure to act on research misconduct. *Lancet* 2000;**356**:2030.
22 Nylenna M, Andersen D, Dahlquist G, Sarvas M, Aakvaag A. Handling of scientific dishonesty in the Nordic countries. *Lancet* 1999;**354**:57–61.

Appendix: Standard operating procedure (SOP) for the handling of suspected fraud/ misconduct

1 Objective

1.1 The objective of this SOP is to set out the procedures and responsibilities for the investigation and management of cases of suspected fraud/misconduct occurring in clinical research.

1.2 An outline of the procedures adopted by the Association of the British Pharmaceutical Industry and the General Medical Council, following company notification, are also covered.

1.3 It should be remembered that whilst all fraud is misconduct, not all misconduct amounts to fraud, only specialist investigation can reach this conclusion.

2 Scope

This SOP covers all cases of suspected fraud/misconduct occurring in clinical research from Phases I–IV and SAMM studies regardless of the type of study. The SOP is also applicable to Medical Research Division studies.

3 Applications

See Table A1.

Table A1. Standard operating procedures: activities and responsibilities.

Activity	Responsibility
Detection of suspected fraud/misconduct	Anyone who handles clinical data or has contact with investigators
Chairing of the initial assessment meeting following discussion of the	Quality Assurance Manager

Table A1. (*continued*)

Activity	Responsibility
original person detecting the fraud/ misconduct with their line manager	
The quarantining of data and adverse drug reactions	Clinical Data Manager
The decision to withhold payments	Medical Adviser/Medical Director
Initiating the site audit	Quality Assurance Manager
Presentation of positive audit data to Managing Director, Chief Executive Officer and Legal Affairs	Medical Director
Production of the Statutory Declaration	Specialist Investigator appointed or Company Lawyer
Liaison with the General Medical Council and formal hearing	Specialist Investigator appointed or Company Lawyer

4 Policy

4.1 It is a requirement of continued employment with this Company that all employees suspecting misconduct report them, as outlined in this SOP.

4.2 It is the policy of this Company that all cases of suspected misconduct confirmed by site audit will be prosecuted.

4.3 The method of prosecution will be through a Statutory Declaration made by the Medical Director of the Company.

4.4 Cases of suspected fraud/misconduct will *normally* be pursued through the ABPI procedure and not through the civil courts.

4.5 Cases of suspected fraud/misconduct not positively confirmed by audit, but where a high index of suspicion remained, will be dealt with at the discretion of the Medical Director/Medical Adviser.

5 Procedure

5.1 Cases of suspected fraud/misconduct, whoever detects them, will be reported to the line manager of the person concerned.

5.2 If the line manager agrees that a *prima facie* case for fraud/misconduct exists, he/she will notify the Clinical Quality Assurance Manager.

5.3 If the line manager does not concur with the reporting person's suspicion, there exists the right for the reporting person to communicate directly with the Quality Assurance Manager to avoid collusion.

5.4 The data will be reviewed at a meeting of the Data Manager, the Quality Assurance Manager, the Project Manager/Medical Adviser, and the reporting person under the chairmanship of the Quality Assurance Manager.

5.5 If this meeting does not believe that there is a *prima facie* case for fraud, a report is issued by the Quality Assurance Manager to the line manager of the reporting person and the reporting person, summarising their reasons for not proceeding. (This process may take five days).

5.6 If a *prima facie* case exists the following activities are initiated:

5.6.1 The Data Manager is responsible for quarantining the data and adverse drug reactions

5.6.2 The Medical Adviser/Medical Director will review the feasibility of withholding payments and notify the Management Information Systems administrator of the decision.

5.6.3 Data verification audit will be initiated by the Quality Assurance Manager.

The type of audit may vary according to the study in question. It should ideally consist of the Quality Assurance Manager together with the Trial Monitor, Medical Director or Medical Adviser. It may, in the case of post-marketing surveillance, be only the Trial Monitor responsible for that area.

5.7 A formal report of the data verification audit is issued. The following activities may then be initiated:

5.7.1 If fraud/misconduct is not confirmed at audit, any further action is at the discretion of the Medical Director/Medical Adviser.

5.7.2 If clinical fraud/misconduct is confirmed at audit a formal report is issued to the Medical Director.

5.8 On receipt of this report the Medical Director will set up a meeting with the Managing Director, the Chief Executive Officer, and a representative of Legal Affairs, and will brief them on the case to date.

This whole procedure, from the first suspicion of fraud/misconduct to the briefing of the Chief Executive Officer will take no more than 25 working days.

5.9 Following the briefing of the senior executives' meeting and assuming a decision to proceed, it is the responsibility of the Medical Director to prepare a Statutory Declaration.

5.10

5.10.1 The Statutory Declaration should be sent to the General Medical Council.

5.10.2 If the preliminary screener at the General Medical Council (GMC) believes that the case should proceed it may be sent to the Preliminary Proceedings Committee under the GMC procedure rules. A decision as to future progress rests with that committee who may:

a) take no further action

b) send a warning letter to the respondent doctor

c) refer to the Health Committee if appropriate

d) refer to the Professional Conduct Committee for a full hearing.

5.10.3 The complainant company will be notified by the GMC as to progress of the case.

5.11 Company Medical Directors are advised to inform the Medical Director of the Association of the British Pharmaceutical Industry of any investigator they suspect of research misconduct. The ABPI Medical Director will be in a position to advise the company on how to proceed.

6 Training

6.1 It is the responsibility of the Company Medical Director to ensure that all those involved with clinical trial activity within the company are appropriately trained to discover and handle any cases of misconduct/fraud. Advice on training programmes is available from the Medical Director of the ABPI.

Index

263